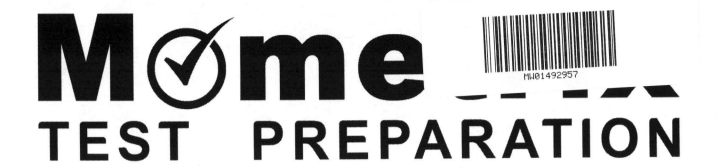

# Mome TEST PREPARATION

## Secrets of the
# General Chairside Assisting Exam
## Study Guide

# DEAR FUTURE EXAM SUCCESS STORY

First of all, **THANK YOU** for purchasing Mometrix study materials!

Second, congratulations! You are one of the few determined test-takers who are committed to doing whatever it takes to excel on your exam. **You have come to the right place.** We developed these study materials with one goal in mind: to deliver you the information you need in a format that's concise and easy to use.

In addition to optimizing your guide for the content of the test, we've outlined our recommended steps for breaking down the preparation process into small, attainable goals so you can make sure you stay on track.

We've also analyzed the entire test-taking process, identifying the most common pitfalls and showing how you can overcome them and be ready for any curveball the test throws you.

Standardized testing is one of the biggest obstacles on your road to success, which only increases the importance of doing well in the high-pressure, high-stakes environment of test day. Your results on this test could have a significant impact on your future, and this guide provides the information and practical advice to help you achieve your full potential on test day.

Your success is our success

**We would love to hear from you!** If you would like to share the story of your exam success or if you have any questions or comments in regard to our products, please contact us at **800-673-8175** or **support@mometrix.com**.

Thanks again for your business and we wish you continued success!

Sincerely,
The Mometrix Test Preparation Team

---

Need more help? Check out our flashcards at:<br>http://mometrixflashcards.com/DANB

# TABLE OF CONTENTS

# Introduction

**Thank you for purchasing this resource**! You have made the choice to prepare yourself for a test that could have a huge impact on your future, and this guide is designed to help you be fully ready for test day. Obviously, it's important to have a solid understanding of the test material, but you also need to be prepared for the unique environment and stressors of the test, so that you can perform to the best of your abilities.

For this purpose, the first section that appears in this guide is the **Secret Keys**. We've devoted countless hours to meticulously researching what works and what doesn't, and we've boiled down our findings to the five most impactful steps you can take to improve your performance on the test. We start at the beginning with study planning and move through the preparation process, all the way to the testing strategies that will help you get the most out of what you know when you're finally sitting in front of the test.

We recommend that you start preparing for your test as far in advance as possible. However, if you've bought this guide as a last-minute study resource and only have a few days before your test, we recommend that you skip over the first two Secret Keys since they address a long-term study plan.

If you struggle with **test anxiety**, we strongly encourage you to check out our recommendations for how you can overcome it. Test anxiety is a formidable foe, but it can be beaten, and we want to make sure you have the tools you need to defeat it.

# Secret Key #1 – Plan Big, Study Small

There's a lot riding on your performance. If you want to ace this test, you're going to need to keep your skills sharp and the material fresh in your mind. You need a plan that lets you review everything you need to know while still fitting in your schedule. We'll break this strategy down into three categories.

## Information Organization

Start with the information you already have: the official test outline. From this, you can make a complete list of all the concepts you need to cover before the test. Organize these concepts into groups that can be studied together, and create a list of any related vocabulary you need to learn so you can brush up on any difficult terms. You'll want to keep this vocabulary list handy once you actually start studying since you may need to add to it along the way.

## Time Management

Once you have your set of study concepts, decide how to spread them out over the time you have left before the test. Break your study plan into small, clear goals so you have a manageable task for each day and know exactly what you're doing. Then just focus on one small step at a time. When you manage your time this way, you don't need to spend hours at a time studying. Studying a small block of content for a short period each day helps you retain information better and avoid stressing over how much you have left to do. You can relax knowing that you have a plan to cover everything in time. In order for this strategy to be effective though, you have to start studying early and stick to your schedule. Avoid the exhaustion and futility that comes from last-minute cramming!

## Study Environment

The environment you study in has a big impact on your learning. Studying in a coffee shop, while probably more enjoyable, is not likely to be as fruitful as studying in a quiet room. It's important to keep distractions to a minimum. You're only planning to study for a short block of time, so make the most of it. Don't pause to check your phone or get up to find a snack. It's also important to **avoid multitasking**. Research has consistently shown that multitasking will make your studying dramatically less effective. Your study area should also be comfortable and well-lit so you don't have the distraction of straining your eyes or sitting on an uncomfortable chair.

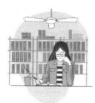 The time of day you study is also important. You want to be rested and alert. Don't wait until just before bedtime. Study when you'll be most likely to comprehend and remember. Even better, if you know what time of day your test will be, set that time aside for study. That way your brain will be used to working on that subject at that specific time and you'll have a better chance of recalling information.

Finally, it can be helpful to team up with others who are studying for the same test. Your actual studying should be done in as isolated an environment as possible, but the work of organizing the information and setting up the study plan can be divided up. In between study sessions, you can discuss with your teammates the concepts that you're all studying and quiz each other on the details. Just be sure that your teammates are as serious about the test as you are. If you find that your study time is being replaced with social time, you might need to find a new team.

# Secret Key #2 – Make Your Studying Count

You're devoting a lot of time and effort to preparing for this test, so you want to be absolutely certain it will pay off. This means doing more than just reading the content and hoping you can remember it on test day. It's important to make every minute of study count. There are two main areas you can focus on to make your studying count.

## Retention

It doesn't matter how much time you study if you can't remember the material. You need to make sure you are retaining the concepts. To check your retention of the information you're learning, try recalling it at later times with minimal prompting. Try carrying around flashcards and glance at one or two from time to time or ask a friend who's also studying for the test to quiz you.

To enhance your retention, look for ways to put the information into practice so that you can apply it rather than simply recalling it. If you're using the information in practical ways, it will be much easier to remember. Similarly, it helps to solidify a concept in your mind if you're not only reading it to yourself but also explaining it to someone else. Ask a friend to let you teach them about a concept you're a little shaky on (or speak aloud to an imaginary audience if necessary). As you try to summarize, define, give examples, and answer your friend's questions, you'll understand the concepts better and they will stay with you longer. Finally, step back for a big picture view and ask yourself how each piece of information fits with the whole subject. When you link the different concepts together and see them working together as a whole, it's easier to remember the individual components.

Finally, practice showing your work on any multi-step problems, even if you're just studying. Writing out each step you take to solve a problem will help solidify the process in your mind, and you'll be more likely to remember it during the test.

## Modality

*Modality* simply refers to the means or method by which you study. Choosing a study modality that fits your own individual learning style is crucial. No two people learn best in exactly the same way, so it's important to know your strengths and use them to your advantage.

For example, if you learn best by visualization, focus on visualizing a concept in your mind and draw an image or a diagram. Try color-coding your notes, illustrating them, or creating symbols that will trigger your mind to recall a learned concept. If you learn best by hearing or discussing information, find a study partner who learns the same way or read aloud to yourself. Think about how to put the information in your own words. Imagine that you are giving a lecture on the topic and record yourself so you can listen to it later.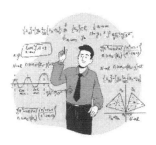

For any learning style, flashcards can be helpful. Organize the information so you can take advantage of spare moments to review. Underline key words or phrases. Use different colors for different categories. Mnemonic devices (such as creating a short list in which every item starts with the same letter) can also help with retention. Find what works best for you and use it to store the information in your mind most effectively and easily.

3

# Secret Key #3 – Practice the Right Way

Your success on test day depends not only on how many hours you put into preparing, but also on whether you prepared the right way. It's good to check along the way to see if your studying is paying off. One of the most effective ways to do this is by taking practice tests to evaluate your progress. Practice tests are useful because they show exactly where you need to improve. Every time you take a practice test, pay special attention to these three groups of questions:

- The questions you got wrong
- The questions you had to guess on, even if you guessed right
- The questions you found difficult or slow to work through

This will show you exactly what your weak areas are, and where you need to devote more study time. Ask yourself why each of these questions gave you trouble. Was it because you didn't understand the material? Was it because you didn't remember the vocabulary? Do you need more repetitions on this type of question to build speed and confidence? Dig into those questions and figure out how you can strengthen your weak areas as you go back to review the material.

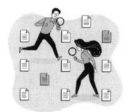 Additionally, many practice tests have a section explaining the answer choices. It can be tempting to read the explanation and think that you now have a good understanding of the concept. However, an explanation likely only covers part of the question's broader context. Even if the explanation makes perfect sense, **go back and investigate** every concept related to the question until you're positive you have a thorough understanding.

As you go along, keep in mind that the practice test is just that: practice. Memorizing these questions and answers will not be very helpful on the actual test because it is unlikely to have any of the same exact questions. If you only know the right answers to the sample questions, you won't be prepared for the real thing. **Study the concepts** until you understand them fully, and then you'll be able to answer any question that shows up on the test.

It's important to wait on the practice tests until you're ready. If you take a test on your first day of study, you may be overwhelmed by the amount of material covered and how much you need to learn. Work up to it gradually.

On test day, you'll need to be prepared for answering questions, managing your time, and using the test-taking strategies you've learned. It's a lot to balance, like a mental marathon that will have a big impact on your future. Like training for a marathon, you'll need to start slowly and work your way up. When test day arrives, you'll be ready.

Start with the strategies you've read in the first two Secret Keys—plan your course and study in the way that works best for you. If you have time, consider using multiple study resources to get different approaches to the same concepts. It can be helpful to see difficult concepts from more than one angle. Then find a good source for practice tests. Many times, the test website will suggest potential study resources or provide sample tests.

4

# Practice Test Strategy

If you're able to find at least three practice tests, we recommend this strategy:

### UNTIMED AND OPEN-BOOK PRACTICE

Take the first test with no time constraints and with your notes and study guide handy. Take your time and focus on applying the strategies you've learned.

### TIMED AND OPEN-BOOK PRACTICE

Take the second practice test open-book as well, but set a timer and practice pacing yourself to finish in time.

### TIMED AND CLOSED-BOOK PRACTICE

Take any other practice tests as if it were test day. Set a timer and put away your study materials. Sit at a table or desk in a quiet room, imagine yourself at the testing center, and answer questions as quickly and accurately as possible.

Keep repeating timed and closed-book tests on a regular basis until you run out of practice tests or it's time for the actual test. Your mind will be ready for the schedule and stress of test day, and you'll be able to focus on recalling the material you've learned.

# Secret Key #4 – Pace Yourself

Once you're fully prepared for the material on the test, your biggest challenge on test day will be managing your time. Just knowing that the clock is ticking can make you panic even if you have plenty of time left. Work on pacing yourself so you can build confidence against the time constraints of the exam. Pacing is a difficult skill to master, especially in a high-pressure environment, so **practice is vital**.

Set time expectations for your pace based on how much time is available. For example, if a section has 60 questions and the time limit is 30 minutes, you know you have to average 30 seconds or less per question in order to answer them all. Although 30 seconds is the hard limit, set 25 seconds per question as your goal, so you reserve extra time to spend on harder questions. When you budget extra time for the harder questions, you no longer have any reason to stress when those questions take longer to answer.

Don't let this time expectation distract you from working through the test at a calm, steady pace, but keep it in mind so you don't spend too much time on any one question. Recognize that taking extra time on one question you don't understand may keep you from answering two that you do understand later in the test. If your time limit for a question is up and you're still not sure of the answer, mark it and move on, and come back to it later if the time and the test format allow. If the testing format doesn't allow you to return to earlier questions, just make an educated guess; then put it out of your mind and move on.

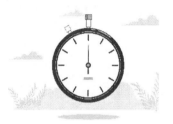

On the easier questions, be careful not to rush. It may seem wise to hurry through them so you have more time for the challenging ones, but it's not worth missing one if you know the concept and just didn't take the time to read the question fully. Work efficiently but make sure you understand the question and have looked at all of the answer choices, since more than one may seem right at first.

Even if you're paying attention to the time, you may find yourself a little behind at some point. You should speed up to get back on track, but do so wisely. Don't panic; just take a few seconds less on each question until you're caught up. Don't guess without thinking, but do look through the answer choices and eliminate any you know are wrong. If you can get down to two choices, it is often worthwhile to guess from those. Once you've chosen an answer, move on and don't dwell on any that you skipped or had to hurry through. If a question was taking too long, chances are it was one of the harder ones, so you weren't as likely to get it right anyway.

On the other hand, if you find yourself getting ahead of schedule, it may be beneficial to slow down a little. The more quickly you work, the more likely you are to make a careless mistake that will affect your score. You've budgeted time for each question, so don't be afraid to spend that time. Practice an efficient but careful pace to get the most out of the time you have.

# Secret Key #5 – Have a Plan for Guessing

When you're taking the test, you may find yourself stuck on a question. Some of the answer choices seem better than others, but you don't see the one answer choice that is obviously correct. What do you do?

The scenario described above is very common, yet most test takers have not effectively prepared for it. Developing and practicing a plan for guessing may be one of the single most effective uses of your time as you get ready for the exam.

In developing your plan for guessing, there are three questions to address:

- When should you start the guessing process?
- How should you narrow down the choices?
- Which answer should you choose?

## When to Start the Guessing Process

Unless your plan for guessing is to select C every time (which, despite its merits, is not what we recommend), you need to leave yourself enough time to apply your answer elimination strategies. Since you have a limited amount of time for each question, that means that if you're going to give yourself the best shot at guessing correctly, you have to decide quickly whether or not you will guess.

Of course, the best-case scenario is that you don't have to guess at all, so first, see if you can answer the question based on your knowledge of the subject and basic reasoning skills. Focus on the key words in the question and try to jog your memory of related topics. Give yourself a chance to bring the knowledge to mind, but once you realize that you don't have (or you can't access) the knowledge you need to answer the question, it's time to start the guessing process.

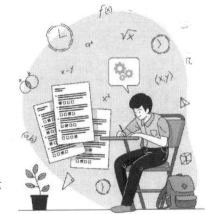

It's almost always better to start the guessing process too early than too late. It only takes a few seconds to remember something and answer the question from knowledge. Carefully eliminating wrong answer choices takes longer. Plus, going through the process of eliminating answer choices can actually help jog your memory.

**Summary**: Start the guessing process as soon as you decide that you can't answer the question based on your knowledge.

# How to Narrow Down the Choices

The next chapter in this book (**Test-Taking Strategies**) includes a wide range of strategies for how to approach questions and how to look for answer choices to eliminate. You will definitely want to read those carefully, practice them, and figure out which ones work best for you. Here though, we're going to address a mindset rather than a particular strategy.

Your odds of guessing an answer correctly depend on how many options you are choosing from.

| Number of options left | 5 | 4 | 3 | 2 | 1 |
|---|---|---|---|---|---|
| Odds of guessing correctly | 20% | 25% | 33% | 50% | 100% |

You can see from this chart just how valuable it is to be able to eliminate incorrect answers and make an educated guess, but there are two things that many test takers do that cause them to miss out on the benefits of guessing:

- Accidentally eliminating the correct answer
- Selecting an answer based on an impression

We'll look at the first one here, and the second one in the next section.

To avoid accidentally eliminating the correct answer, we recommend a thought exercise called **the $5 challenge**. In this challenge, you only eliminate an answer choice from contention if you are willing to bet $5 on it being wrong. Why $5? Five dollars is a small but not insignificant amount of money. It's an amount you could afford to lose but wouldn't want to throw away. And while losing

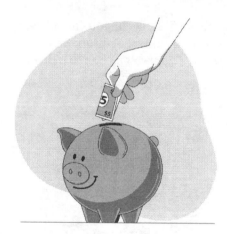

$5 once might not hurt too much, doing it twenty times will set you back $100. In the same way, each small decision you make—eliminating a choice here, guessing on a question there—won't by itself impact your score very much, but when you put them all together, they can make a big difference. By holding each answer choice elimination decision to a higher standard, you can reduce the risk of accidentally eliminating the correct answer.

The $5 challenge can also be applied in a positive sense: If you are willing to bet $5 that an answer choice *is* correct, go ahead and mark it as correct.

**Summary**: Only eliminate an answer choice if you are willing to bet $5 that it is wrong.

8

# Which Answer to Choose

You're taking the test. You've run into a hard question and decided you'll have to guess. You've eliminated all the answer choices you're willing to bet $5 on. Now you have to pick an answer. Why do we even need to talk about this? Why can't you just pick whichever one you feel like when the time comes?

The answer to these questions is that if you don't come into the test with a plan, you'll rely on your impression to select an answer choice, and if you do that, you risk falling into a trap. The test writers know that everyone who takes their test will be guessing on some of the questions, so they intentionally write wrong answer choices to seem plausible. You still have to pick an answer though, and if the wrong answer choices are designed to look right, how can you ever be sure that you're not falling for their trap? The best solution we've found to this dilemma is to take the decision out of your hands entirely. Here is the process we recommend:

**Once you've eliminated any choices that you are confident (willing to bet $5) are wrong, select the first remaining choice as your answer.**

Whether you choose to select the first remaining choice, the second, or the last, the important thing is that you use some preselected standard. Using this approach guarantees that you will not be enticed into selecting an answer choice that looks right, because you are not basing your decision on how the answer choices look.

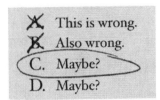

This is not meant to make you question your knowledge. Instead, it is to help you recognize the difference between your knowledge and your impressions. There's a huge difference between thinking an answer is right because of what you know, and thinking an answer is right because it looks or sounds like it should be right.

**Summary**: To ensure that your selection is appropriately random, make a predetermined selection from among all answer choices you have not eliminated.

# Test-Taking Strategies

This section contains a list of test-taking strategies that you may find helpful as you work through the test. By taking what you know and applying logical thought, you can maximize your chances of answering any question correctly!

It is very important to realize that every question is different and every person is different: no single strategy will work on every question, and no single strategy will work for every person. That's why we've included all of them here, so you can try them out and determine which ones work best for different types of questions and which ones work best for you.

## Question Strategies

### ☑ READ CAREFULLY

Read the question and the answer choices carefully. Don't miss the question because you misread the terms. You have plenty of time to read each question thoroughly and make sure you understand what is being asked. Yet a happy medium must be attained, so don't waste too much time. You must read carefully and efficiently.

### ☑ CONTEXTUAL CLUES

Look for contextual clues. If the question includes a word you are not familiar with, look at the immediate context for some indication of what the word might mean. Contextual clues can often give you all the information you need to decipher the meaning of an unfamiliar word. Even if you can't determine the meaning, you may be able to narrow down the possibilities enough to make a solid guess at the answer to the question.

### ☑ PREFIXES

If you're having trouble with a word in the question or answer choices, try dissecting it. Take advantage of every clue that the word might include. Prefixes can be a huge help. Usually, they allow you to determine a basic meaning. *Pre-* means before, *post-* means after, *pro-* is positive, *de-* is negative. From prefixes, you can get an idea of the general meaning of the word and try to put it into context.

### ☑ HEDGE WORDS

Watch out for critical hedge words, such as *likely, may, can, sometimes, often, almost, mostly, usually, generally, rarely,* and *sometimes*. Question writers insert these hedge phrases to cover every possibility. Often an answer choice will be wrong simply because it leaves no room for exception. Be on guard for answer choices that have definitive words such as *exactly* and *always*.

### ☑ SWITCHBACK WORDS

Stay alert for *switchbacks*. These are the words and phrases frequently used to alert you to shifts in thought. The most common switchback words are *but, although,* and *however*. Others include *nevertheless, on the other hand, even though, while, in spite of, despite,* and *regardless of*. Switchback words are important to catch because they can change the direction of the question or an answer choice.

## ⊘ FACE VALUE

When in doubt, use common sense. Accept the situation in the problem at face value. Don't read too much into it. These problems will not require you to make wild assumptions. If you have to go beyond creativity and warp time or space in order to have an answer choice fit the question, then you should move on and consider the other answer choices. These are normal problems rooted in reality. The applicable relationship or explanation may not be readily apparent, but it is there for you to figure out. Use your common sense to interpret anything that isn't clear.

# Answer Choice Strategies

## ⊘ ANSWER SELECTION

The most thorough way to pick an answer choice is to identify and eliminate wrong answers until only one is left, then confirm it is the correct answer. Sometimes an answer choice may immediately seem right, but be careful. The test writers will usually put more than one reasonable answer choice on each question, so take a second to read all of them and make sure that the other choices are not equally obvious. As long as you have time left, it is better to read every answer choice than to pick the first one that looks right without checking the others.

## ⊘ ANSWER CHOICE FAMILIES

An answer choice family consists of two (in rare cases, three) answer choices that are very similar in construction and cannot all be true at the same time. If you see two answer choices that are direct opposites or parallels, one of them is usually the correct answer. For instance, if one answer choice says that quantity $x$ increases and another either says that quantity $x$ decreases (opposite) or says that quantity $y$ increases (parallel), then those answer choices would fall into the same family. An answer choice that doesn't match the construction of the answer choice family is more likely to be incorrect. Most questions will not have answer choice families, but when they do appear, you should be prepared to recognize them.

## ⊘ ELIMINATE ANSWERS

Eliminate answer choices as soon as you realize they are wrong, but make sure you consider all possibilities. If you are eliminating answer choices and realize that the last one you are left with is also wrong, don't panic. Start over and consider each choice again. There may be something you missed the first time that you will realize on the second pass.

## ⊘ AVOID FACT TRAPS

Don't be distracted by an answer choice that is factually true but doesn't answer the question. You are looking for the choice that answers the question. Stay focused on what the question is asking for so you don't accidentally pick an answer that is true but incorrect. Always go back to the question and make sure the answer choice you've selected actually answers the question and is not merely a true statement.

## ⊘ EXTREME STATEMENTS

In general, you should avoid answers that put forth extreme actions as standard practice or proclaim controversial ideas as established fact. An answer choice that states the "process should be used in certain situations, if..." is much more likely to be correct than one that states the "process should be discontinued completely." The first is a calm rational statement and doesn't even make a definitive, uncompromising stance, using a hedge word *if* to provide wiggle room, whereas the second choice is far more extreme.

## ⊘ Benchmark

As you read through the answer choices and you come across one that seems to answer the question well, mentally select that answer choice. This is not your final answer, but it's the one that will help you evaluate the other answer choices. The one that you selected is your benchmark or standard for judging each of the other answer choices. Every other answer choice must be compared to your benchmark. That choice is correct until proven otherwise by another answer choice beating it. If you find a better answer, then that one becomes your new benchmark. Once you've decided that no other choice answers the question as well as your benchmark, you have your final answer.

## ⊘ Predict the Answer

Before you even start looking at the answer choices, it is often best to try to predict the answer. When you come up with the answer on your own, it is easier to avoid distractions and traps because you will know exactly what to look for. The right answer choice is unlikely to be word-for-word what you came up with, but it should be a close match. Even if you are confident that you have the right answer, you should still take the time to read each option before moving on.

# General Strategies

## ⊘ Tough Questions

If you are stumped on a problem or it appears too hard or too difficult, don't waste time. Move on! Remember though, if you can quickly check for obviously incorrect answer choices, your chances of guessing correctly are greatly improved. Before you completely give up, at least try to knock out a couple of possible answers. Eliminate what you can and then guess at the remaining answer choices before moving on.

## ⊘ Check Your Work

Since you will probably not know every term listed and the answer to every question, it is important that you get credit for the ones that you do know. Don't miss any questions through careless mistakes. If at all possible, try to take a second to look back over your answer selection and make sure you've selected the correct answer choice and haven't made a costly careless mistake (such as marking an answer choice that you didn't mean to mark). This quick double check should more than pay for itself in caught mistakes for the time it costs.

## ⊘ Pace Yourself

It's easy to be overwhelmed when you're looking at a page full of questions; your mind is confused and full of random thoughts, and the clock is ticking down faster than you would like. Calm down and maintain the pace that you have set for yourself. Especially as you get down to the last few minutes of the test, don't let the small numbers on the clock make you panic. As long as you are on track by monitoring your pace, you are guaranteed to have time for each question.

## ⊘ Don't Rush

It is very easy to make errors when you are in a hurry. Maintaining a fast pace in answering questions is pointless if it makes you miss questions that you would have gotten right otherwise. Test writers like to include distracting information and wrong answers that seem right. Taking a little extra time to avoid careless mistakes can make all the difference in your test score. Find a pace that allows you to be confident in the answers that you select.

12

## ⊘ Keep Moving

Panicking will not help you pass the test, so do your best to stay calm and keep moving. Taking deep breaths and going through the answer elimination steps you practiced can help to break through a stress barrier and keep your pace.

# Final Notes

The combination of a solid foundation of content knowledge and the confidence that comes from practicing your plan for applying that knowledge is the key to maximizing your performance on test day. As your foundation of content knowledge is built up and strengthened, you'll find that the strategies included in this chapter become more and more effective in helping you quickly sift through the distractions and traps of the test to isolate the correct answer.

Now that you're preparing to move forward into the test content chapters of this book, be sure to keep your goal in mind. As you read, think about how you will be able to apply this information on the test. If you've already seen sample questions for the test and you have an idea of the question format and style, try to come up with questions of your own that you can answer based on what you're reading. This will give you valuable practice applying your knowledge in the same ways you can expect to on test day.

**Good luck and good studying!**

14

# Patient Preparation and Documentation

## Preliminary Physical Exam

### CHIEF COMPLAINT

The **chief complaint** is the reason the patient has come to the appointment. This is in the patient's own words and is often the first part of the documentation in the dental record for a specific visit. It is often abbreviated as "CC" for documentation purposes.

Examples of the chief complaint as part of the assessment include "tooth pain" or "jaw pain." More information is sometimes documented under the chief complaint section if the patient offers it as part of the reason they are being seen. Examples include "I have a cavity that has been bothering me for a month" or "I think I have an infection in a tooth on the left lower side." More information can be gathered and documented about the presenting problem, but the chief complaint should be the reason the patient is there in their own words. Often, the chief complaint is gathered at the time the appointment is made, but this should be verified during the patient's initial assessment at the office.

### REVIEWING AND UPDATING PATIENT'S HEALTH AND DENTAL HISTORY

The **patient's health and dental histories** should be updated at least once per year, or whenever there is a change in their medical or dental health. Best practice is to ask the patient if there are any changes or updates to their medical or dental history at every appointment. This information can usually be provided by the patient themselves, if they are an adult. For minors, a parent or legal guardian should provide any updated health information for the dental chart.

It is important to update health information in a patient's dental record because there are many systemic illnesses, and medications, that may affect dental health. For example, patients with heart valve disease will require prophylactic antibiotics before dental procedures in order to decrease the risk of developing cardiac complications if a dental infection should occur. Patients with a seizure disorder may be placed on a medication called Dilantin (phenytoin), which can cause overgrowth of the gums. Updating the patient's medical and dental history is imperative to prevent any potential complications that can arise from dental care, whether it is routine preventive care or more complicated dental surgical procedures.

### PERIODONTAL EXAMINATION

A **periodontal examination** consists of the history, radiographs, examination, measurements, charting, and assessment and scaling by the dentist. Good radiographs can show evidence of periodontal disease. Examination of the teeth includes assessment of tooth mobility with two instruments, inspection of the gingivae and supporting structures, and looking for and probing periodontal pockets. Periodontal probes standardized in millimeters are used to measure depths of six surfaces, the facial, lingual, distofacial, distolingual, mesiofacial and mesiolingual. The dental assistant logs the deepest pockets on the periodontal chart, along with pocket depths, furcations, mobility, exudates, and gingival recession. The dentist uses explorers to find calculus and assess the root, straight or curved scalers to get rid of supragingival calculus, and less blunt curettes to remove subgingival calculus.

### EXTERNAL CLINICAL EVALUATION

For the **external clinical evaluation,** scrutinize the patient discreetly as he/she enters the room for indicators of abuse, nutrition issues, poor health, and aging. Focus on these issues that impact

15

dental or orthodontic care: Exaggerated facial asymmetry; swelling (edema); speech problems; abnormal lip smacking; mouth breathing; and thumb sucking. Examine the lips for cracking or parching from dry mouth (xerostomia), which indicates underlying disease (e.g., thrush, vitamin deficiency, hypothyroidism, autoimmune diseases, or psychiatric drug use). Examine the smile line where the lips meet, the peripheral vermillion borderline, and the lip corners or commissures. Ask the patient to close his or her lips. Palpate the mandible and external floor of the mouth externally. Ask the patient to turn his or her head to the side. Feel the cervical lymph nodes between the ear and collarbone. To inspect the patient's temporomandibular joint (TMJ) externally, sit behind the patient. Palpate the tragus in front of the ear as the patient opens and closes his or her mouth. Listen for clicking (crepitus). Watch for snagging. Ask the patient if he/she feels pain.

## INTERNAL CLINICAL EVALUATION

A certified dental or orthodontic assistant can legally perform both the external and internal clinical evaluation in most states. After examining the patient extraorally, perform an **internal oral examination.** Note mouth wounds, abscessed teeth, and abnormal mucosa colorations. Hold the mandible in one hand. Palpate the underside of the tongue and the floor of the mouth. Stand behind the patient. Examine the oral mucosa and frenum (fold) by pulling the lips outward. Use a mouth mirror to inspect the buccal (cheek) area and the tongue. Use gauze to pull the tongue to the side and upward for better vision. Instruct the patient to say "ah." Inspect the entrance to the throat and the oropharynx. In addition, the dentist uses a hand instrument to prod the hard surface of every tooth, and the assistant notes any findings in the patient's record.

## NORMAL OCCLUSION AND FACIAL PROFILES

Occlusion is the relationship between upper and lower teeth when the mouth is closed. In **normal occlusion**, teeth in both dental arches are in maximum contact, without rotation or nonstandard spacing. The front teeth in the maxillary arch overlap the incisal edge of those in the mandible slightly, by about 2 millimeters. The maxillary posterior teeth are positioned one cusp further back than the mandibular posterior ones. Lastly, the mesial buccal cusp of the first permanent molar in the upper arch is in contact with the buccal groove of the first molar in the mandible. Normal occlusion should give a mesognathic **facial profile**, a straight line between jaws with only a slight projection of the mandible, relative to the upper part of the face.

## FACIAL LANDMARKS

The dentist should be aware of the following **landmarks of the face** and **oral cavity** during examination, in order to recognize and note any abnormalities:

- The first facial landmark is the *outside edge or ala of the nose.*
- Extending from the nose to the corner of the mouth is the *naso-labial groove.*
- The *philtrum* is the hollow between the bottom of the nose and the center of the upper lip.
- *Lips have four landmarks:* (1) the vermillion zone, the entire reddish part of the lips, (2) the vermillion border surrounding it, (3) the tubercle of the lip, the slight protrusion in the center of the upper lip, and (4) the labial commissures, the corners of the mouth. The lip vermillion zone is highly vascularized, which makes it pink or red in a healthy person, and blue in a cold, hypoxic, or dead person.
- The final facial landmark is the *labio-mental groove*, a horizontal depression in the middle between the lips and chin.

## NORMAL VALUES FOR VITAL SIGNS

### Temperature:

- Ideal 98.6 °F (37 °C)
- Normal Range 97.8-99 °F (36.5-37.2 °C); lowest in the morning.
- Hypothermia <95 °F (<35 °C) from cold exposure or antipyretics.
- Pyrexia >98.6 °F oral or >99.8 °F rectal; use Tylenol for children and Aspirin for adults.
- Hyperpyrexia 107.6 °F (>42 °C); use cold packs.

### Pulse:

- Normal adult 60-100 beats/min. with a normal sinus rhythm.
- Females beat faster than males.
- Children beat faster (90 to 120 and neonates 144 beats/min.).

>100 bpm in adults is tachycardia.

<50 bpm in adults is bradycardia. Abnormal rhythm is arrhythmia.

### Respiration:

- Normal adult 12-20 per min.
- Children breathe faster (neonates 30-60 per min.).
- Tachypnea is >20 breaths per minute. Bradypnea is < 12 bpm.

### Blood Pressure:

- Upper normal adult 120/80 mm/Hg
- Hypertension 140/90 mm/Hg
- Hypotension 90/50 mm/Hg

### Pain*:

- Pain absent
- Responsive to pain stimulus

* Optional, used to monitor patient during procedure and when the patient recovers from anesthesia

## TAKING PATIENT'S TEMPERATURE, PULSE, AND RESPIRATION

When **taking a patient's vitals,** first the GCA must identify him/herself and explain what they are going to do. Place a clean oral digital thermometer under the patient's tongue, and ask them to close their mouth for the duration of the measurement. Respiration rate indicates efficiency of oxygen intake and carbon dioxide output. Watch the patient's chest rise and fall. One respiration consists of an inhalation followed by an exhalation. Count respirations for 1 minute while holding the radial pulse (inner wrist on thumb side) with the fingertips, so the patient does not hold his or her breath. Do not feel a pulse with the thumb.

Record a baseline at the preliminary exam. Update TPR at subsequent visits. Document immediately, before the visit concludes. If the patient has no arms or the radial pulse cannot be felt, then palpate one of these pulses: Carotid (neck groove beside trachea), brachial (antecubitum below elbow bend), or temporal (depression between eyebrow and ear).

17

## BLOOD PRESSURE MEASUREMENT

**Blood pressure (BP)** is controlled by the hypothalamus, medulla oblongata, and kidney. Pain, exercise, and fear increase blood pressure. Use either a stethoscope and a sphygmomanometer or an automated BP clip to measure BP. A thin adult needs a pediatric cuff. Use a thigh cuff on an obese patient's arm. A normal adult male's BP is 120/80 mm/Hg. Small women and children have lower blood pressures. Elders have higher blood pressure. *Hypotension* (low blood pressure) is below 90/50 mm/Hg. Hypotension leads to dizziness and fainting. *Hypertension* (high blood pressure) is above 140/90 mm/Hg. Hypertension leads to stroke and heart disease. The first Korotkoff sound heard ("lub") is the systole, when the heart contracts to pump oxygenated blood to the arteries from the left chamber of the heart. The second sound ("dub") is the diastole, when the heart relaxes as its right side fills with blood for subsequent oxygenation. BP is the ratio of systolic to diastolic pressure.

## BENIGN ORAL TUMORS

**Oral tumors** are called neoplasms. Benign tumors are not cancerous, but can still cause pain, deformity, and loss of normal use. Some benign tumors have the potential for malignancy:

- *Squamous papillomae* are benign tumors that develop after human papilloma virus (HPV) infections, usually types 6 and 11. Projections of squamous epithelial tissue can be surgically removed.
- *Fibromas* are benign areas of hyperplasia; they present as pink, even, dome-shaped lesions, generally on the buccal surface.
- *Lichen planus* looks like a flattened, deep reed or violet bump. Often, lichen planus is found on the patient's leg or ankle. In the mouth, the buccal mucosa is usually involved, and lines know as Wickham's striae may be seen. The patient usually has soreness while eating. The dentist usually prescribes topical steroids. Its malignant potential is unclear.

## ORAL LESIONS THAT RIDE SURFACE FLATS OF ORAL MUCOSA

The types of **oral lesions** observable on the surface flats of the oral mucosa include macules, ecchymosis, patches, petechiae, purpura, granulomas, neoplasms and nodules. The latter three may also present above the surface of the oral mucosa.

- *Macules* are spots and patches are irregular areas that differ in texture and/or color from their surroundings. An example is white thrush, yeast that colonizes patients with depressed immune systems.
- *Ecchymosis* is bruised tissue.
- Pinpoint hemorrhaging is *petechiae*.
- *Purpura* is small red or purple spots, which includes tiny petechiae, and larger areas of discoloration up to an inch in diameter, such as ecchymosis.
- *Neoplasms* are tumorous growths, either benign (noncancerous) or malignant (cancerous). The dentist refers the patient with a neoplasm to an M.D. for investigation.
- A *granuloma* is one type of neoplasm, in which chronic inflammation produces an area of granulation tissue.
- *Nodules* are small protuberances of either hard or soft tissue.

## SHALLOW LESIONS OBSERVED ON ORAL MUCOSA

**Shallow lesions** that appear on the **surface of the oral mucosa** include blisters, bullas, pustules, vesicles, papules, plaques, and hematomas. Shallow lesions are significant because they may be contagious, are painful, and can prevent the patient from obtaining proper nutrition.

- *Blisters* are thin-walled, fluid-filled sacs resulting from friction or viral diseases. Fluid accumulation occurs when blood vessels leak following trauma. Vesicles, bullas, and pustules are all variations of blisters.
- *Vesicles* are small blisters filled with fluid or gas and usually come from herpes or Varicella.
- *Bullae* are larger, with diameters larger than 0.5 inch.
- *Pustules* are infected blisters containing dead white cells and bacteria as pus.
- *Hematomas* are reddish lesions containing a semi-solid mass of blood from a ruptured blood vessel; hematomas commonly appear after application of oral anesthetic.
- A *plaque* is any elevated (or level) lesion in the oral mucosa.

## DEEP LESIONS OBSERVED UNDERNEATH SURFACE OF ORAL MUCOSA

**Deep lesions** that appear **underneath the surface of the oral mucosa** include abscesses, cysts, ulcers and erosions.

- *Abscesses* are pus-filled cavities resulting from bacterial infection and inflammation in the oral cavity. Most abscesses appear near the apex of the tooth or in the periodontal area. They require high dose antibiotic treatment (usually penicillin) to avoid bone loss, septicemia, and possible heart, kidney, and brain infection.
- *Cysts* are thick-walled cavities that contain fluid or a semi-solid, fluid mixture. Cyst formation usually occurs from duct blockage, but can result from other diseases.
- *Ulcers* occur when mucous membranes are damaged. Ulcers are reddened, painful, open sores.
- *Erosions* are indentations left after trauma; they have red and tender borders.

## PHYSICAL AGENTS THAT CAUSE ORAL LESIONS

Oral lesions can be **caused by physical agents** such as dental procedures, radiation injury, or trauma, which can be self-induced. Incorrect use of dental instruments can tear or bruise the oral mucosa. Incorrect removal of cotton rolls, used to dry tissue, can induce ulcers in the gums. Improperly fitted or worn dentures can cause ulcers. Eventually, folds of extra tissue (hyperplasia) form. The palate develops red, swollen lumps. Particles of silver amalgam, used to fill caries, can catch in tissue and discolor it blue or gray, but an amalgam tattoo poses no health issue. Excess radiation therapy for head and neck cancer damages the teeth roots or ulcerates the target area. Self-induced traumas to the oral cavity include biting the inside of the cheek or contact with a dull object, such as mouth jewelry in piercings. Ask the patient to remove mouth jewelry before imaging.

## HORMONAL CHANGES AND ORAL LESIONS

All of the below **hormonal changes** can result in bleeding at the gum unless good oral hygiene is maintained:

- About 1 in 20 pregnant women develops *pregnancy gingivitis*, in which the gum tissues become inflated and inflamed. Occasionally, tumors develop. Pregnancy gingivitis should subside when hormone levels return to normal.

- Another type of lesion often found in pregnant women is *pyogenic granuloma*. However, it can also affect nonpregnant women and men. Pyogenic granuloma is a rapidly growing, reddened, vascular mass of granulation tissue. It results from a combination of hormonal changes and local irritation.
- *Gingival swelling* can also occur during the hormonal changes associated with puberty, primarily in girls. Once hormonal balance is restored, the gingival enlargement should subside.

## ORAL LESIONS ASSOCIATED WITH HIV/AIDS

**Human immunodeficiency virus (HIV)** suppresses the immune response of acquired immunodeficiency syndrome (AIDS) patients, so they are susceptible to opportunistic infections unusual for adults in their prime. For example, oral thrush (Candida albicans) usually affects nursing babies, and Kaposi's sarcoma usually affects elderly Mediterranean men. HIV infection is transmissible by blood and is incurable, so wearing PPE is important. Good dental hygiene is imperative for AIDS patients because they are especially vulnerable to periodontal lesions due to bacterial and fungal infections. Chemotherapy or long-term antibiotic use trigger Candida in the oral mucosa. Assess for thick, white lines superimposed over red, inflamed areas, particularly on the tongue or cheeks. Give antifungals, like Nystatin. HIV-positive patients often have hairy leukoplakia or white patterns near the edges of the tongue. The vascular malignancy Kaposi's sarcoma presents as scattered bluish-purple lesions on the palate, nose, and arms that bleed. Low-dose radiation and/or chemotherapy are indicated.

## APHTHOUS ULCERS

**Aphthous ulcers** are canker sores, painful oral ulcerations of unknown origin. Aphthous ulcers have lesions with yellow centers encircled by red halos. The yellow center is actually necrosis of epithelial cells. Aphthous ulcers do not appear to be contagious. Causative agents have not been positively identified. However, Streptococci are often been found in the ulcers. Other factors that promote aphthous ulcer formation are stress, hormonal changes, and food allergies. Aphthous ulcers recur periodically when the patient experiences one of these triggers. Aphthous ulcers typically persist for 10 to 14 days. Sooth aphthous ulcers with topical anesthetics, e.g., Anbesol. Postpone oral procedures during exacerbations, as aphthous ulcers are very painful.

## ORAL INFLAMMATION

**Inflammation** is the body's reaction to infection, allergy, or injury. Inflammation is characterized by redness, heat, swelling, and pain. Inflammation occurs because an injury, allergy, or disease causes immune cells to release histamine into the area. Histamine increases blood flow, manifesting as redness and heat. Histamine makes vessels leaky. Excess blood seeps from the capillaries into surrounding tissues, causing distension. Nearby nerve receptors register inflammation as pain. White blood cells (leukocytes) are recruited to the site to kill microorganisms. Fibrous connective tissue surrounds the area in a web. Be attuned to the signs and symptoms of inflammation because they represent an underlying disease process. Oral inflammation can be observed as a variety of lesions on the mucosal surface.

## MISCELLANEOUS DISORDERS OF ORAL CAVITY

One of the most common **miscellaneous disorders of the oral cavity** is *geographic tongue*, in which smooth red patches bounded by yellow or white edges cover the back and sides of the tongue and filiform papillae (hairy extensions) are missing. Geographic tongue does not hurt and requires no intervention.

*Acute necrotizing ulcerative gingivitis (ANUG)* often occurs in teenagers and young adults and is infectious. ANUG is characterized by oral cavity pain, infection, bleeding, and a foul odor. Clean and debride the affected area. Give antibiotics and hot water rinses.

A *mucocele* is a mucus filled bump inside the mouth closed by trauma or obstruction of a salivary duct. The dentist may lance the mucocele to drain accumulated fluid.

*Varix* is weakened and distended blood vessels in the mouth.

*Bell's palsy* causes drooping features because of temporary paralysis of facial muscles on one side.

## DEVELOPMENTAL ABNORMALITIES ON TONGUE OR IN ORAL CAVITY

One of the most **common developmental abnormalities involving the tongue** is fissured tongue, in which the tongue surface is deeply grooved and sometimes asymmetrical (unevenly shaped). A bifid tongue occurs when the sides of the front of the tongue do not fuse fully, and a tip of muscle is exposed at the end of the tongue. Usually, both of these conditions are left untreated. Ankyloglossia is the connection of the lingual frenulum close to the tip of the tongue, impeding its movement, and preventing the speaker from making certain sounds clearly. It can be corrected with a simple surgical procedure that cuts the frenulum. The vast majority of affected patients also have an abnormality called Fordyce's spots or granules, sebaceous oil glands close to surface epithelia in the oral mucosa.

## CONGENITAL OR EARLY DEVELOPMENTAL ABNORMALITIES IN ORAL CAVITY

**Congenital conditions** are genetically inherited states. Nine common congenital abnormalities found in the oral cavity include:

- Cleft lip (hare lip) or cleft palate.
- Unusually large teeth (macrodontia).
- Unusually small teeth (microdontia) often associated with Down syndrome or congenital heart disease. Amelogenesis imperfecta and dentinogenesis imperfect, hereditary conditions thinning the enamel, discoloring it (amelogenesis), or making it opalescent (dentinogenesis) and prone to caries and enamel wear.
- Congenitally missing teeth (anodontia).
- Extra teeth (supernumerary), present at birth and quickly shed
- Fusion of two or more teeth.
- Ankylosis, the fusion of a tooth, cementum, or dentin to the alveolar bone.
- Gemination, in which a tooth bud cannot fully divide.
- Twinning, the development of two distinct teeth from one tooth bud.

## CLEFT LIP AND CLEFT PALATE

Both cleft lip and cleft palate are developmental failures of tissues in the oral cavity to fuse properly. **Cleft lip** occurs when maxillary processes in the head do not fuse with the medial nasal process, resulting in a notching or more pronounced indentation from the lip to nostril. It can be unilateral (on one side) or bilateral (on both sides). **Cleft palate** occurs when the palatal shelves do not fuse with the primary palate or each other. It can be found alone or in combination with cleft lip. There are different types of cleft palate, depending on the fusion failure. The least severe is cleft uvula, in which only the uvular flap at the back of the soft palate fails to fuse. More serious variations include: Bilateral cleft of the secondary palate; bilateral cleft lip, alveolar process, and primary palate; bilateral cleft of the lip, alveolar process and both primary and secondary palates; unilateral cleft lip, primary palate, and alveolar process. The infant requires maxillofacial surgery.

## ORAL TORI AND EXOSTOSES

**Oral tori** are benign, boney extensions into the oral cavity covered with fine layers of tissue. Extensions developing from the maxillary hard palate are called torus palatinus. They occur in about 20% of adults and are usually near the midline. Torus mandibularis, outgrowths in canine or premolar areas of the mandible, are less common but more bothersome, because food fragments imbed there. Both oral tori can cause tenderness during oral radiography. They should be surgically excised if dental appliances are necessary.

**Exostosis** is the swelling or nodular outgrowth of the lamella bone on the facial side of the maxillary or mandibular palates. It is very similar to oral tori.

## SIGNS OF PERIODONTAL DISEASES

**Periodontal diseases** involve the periodontium, the tissue that surrounds and holds up the teeth. Periodontal diseases can lead to tooth loss through lack of support. Most periodontal disease starts as inflammation resulting from the buildup of plaque, bacterial colonies sticking to teeth or areas of the gingivae. Mineralized plaque on teeth is called dental calculus. Caries can develop from plaque when sugars are converted into acids by the bacteria. Periodontal disease can also result from hormonal disturbances or other oral problems. Risk factors include: Diabetes; poor oral hygiene; osteoporosis; stress; certain medications; HIV/AIDS; irritation from dental appliances; and malocclusion. One type of periodontal disease involves the gums (gingivae); the presence of inflamed and bleeding gums is gingivitis. If the bacterial infection spreads to the underlying supporting alveolar bone, periodontitis results.

## MALOCCLUSION
### ANGLE'S CLASSIFICATIONS

Malocclusion is any divergence from normal occlusion. **Angle's classifications** are used most often to describe three basic types of malocclusion:

- *Neutroclusion (Class I)*, in which occlusion is essentially normal, except that individual or groups of teeth are out of position and the facial profile is still mesognathic.
- *Distoclusion (Class II)*, in which the buccal groove of the mandibular first permanent molar is behind the mesiobuccal cusp of the corresponding maxillary molar. Distoclusion can be Division 1 or 2, due to either outward protrusion of the maxillary teeth or backward sloping of the mandibular teeth. Both produce a retrognathic facial profile, where one or both jaws are recessed.
- *Mesioclusion (Class III)*, in which the buccal groove of the mandibular first permanent molar is mesial to the mesiobuccal cusp of the corresponding maxillary molar. The facial profile is prognathic, meaning the jaws project beyond the upper part of the face.

### CAUSES

Malocclusion is **caused** by one of three factors:

- *Inherited genetic factors* can contribute to formation of extra or supernumerary teeth, missing teeth, atypical relationships between the jaws, or between teeth and the jaw, and deviations such as cleft palate.
- *Exposure to systemic diseases or nutritional deficiencies* during the formative years can interrupt the normal developmental pattern of dentition.
- *Particular habits or localized trauma* can produce malocclusion. These include mouth breathing, thumb or tongue sucking, thrusting of the tongue, nail biting, and bruxism. Bruxism is the unconscious grinding of teeth during sleep or stressful situations.

## MALPOSITION OF INDIVIDUAL TEETH

**Individual teeth** can exhibit the following variations and contribute to malocclusion:

- Teeth that are mesial, distal, or lingual to their normal position are examples of mesioversion, distoversion and linguoversion, respectively.
- Torsoversion is the rotation or turning of a tooth from the expected position.
- Buccoversion or labioversion is the inclination of a tooth toward the cheek or lip. If the crown of an individual tooth is outside the normal line of occlusion, it exhibits either supraversion (above) or infraversion (below).
- Finally, a tooth may appear in the wrong position or order of the dental arch, a variation called transversion or transposition.

## ABNORMAL BITES

A **cross-bite** is an atypical relationship between single teeth or groups of teeth in one dental arch, relative to the other. With a cross-bite involving anterior teeth, the incisors in the maxilla are lingual to the opposing ones in the mandible. Posterior cross-bite presents similarly, with maxillary back teeth closer to the tongue than the mandibular teeth, the opposite of that expected with a normal bite.

An **edge-edge bite** is one in which the incisal surfaces of teeth in both arches converge.

An **end-to-end bite** occurs between posterior teeth whose cusps meet.

An **open bite** is one in which there is a lack of occlusion between the mandibular and maxillary teeth.

## OVERBITE AND OVERJET

Overbite and overjet are two types of malposition between groups of teeth that result in malocclusion. Both are teeth overlaps.

- An **overbite** is a greater than normal vertical overlap between anterior maxillary and mandibular teeth. An overbite means the upper incisors extend over more than one-third of the front teeth in the mandible.
- An **overjet** is horizontal overlap, with an unusually large horizontal distance between the outer surface of the anterior mandibular teeth and the inner face of the maxillary anterior teeth.
- A person can also have an **underjet**, where the front teeth in the mandible project significantly in front of the maxillary anterior teeth.

## TMJ DYSFUNCTION

**TMJ (temporomandibular joint) dysfunction** is lack of coordination in the structures associated with the TMJ. It can present as: Pain near the ear, often extending into the face; soreness in the chewing muscles; popping or clicking noises when opening or closing the mouth; crepitus (grating); tinnitus (ringing in the ears); headache or neck pain; inability to adequately open the mouth (trismus) or move the lower jaw.

**Diagnosis of TMJ dysfunction** or disease is based on a combination of medical and dental history, physical examination, evaluation by tomographic radiography or magnetic resonance imaging, and casts of the teeth to replicate the movements of the jaws. In particular, ask the patient about grinding or clamping the teeth, bite issues, injuries, diseases, and stress when taking the history.

The clinician examines the area by palpation, takes note of characteristic sounds while the jaw is opened and closed, and quantifies how wide the patient can open his or her mouth.

## TREATMENT

Some **treatment options for TMJ dysfunction** are relatively minor, such as: Stress management; rotating heat and cold application; resting the jaw; and NSAID pain relievers, muscle relaxants, antibiotics, mood enhancers, and anti-anxiety drugs. Physiotherapy and massage are often helpful. If minor treatments do not alleviate pain, the dentist progresses to steroid injections into the intra-articular area. The dentist may apply occlusal splints to alleviate spasms or pressure. Often, TMJ disorders are treatable with orthodontia and other restoration. For extreme cases that do not respond to conventional treatments, several types of surgery can be attempted by a maxillofacial surgeon. TMJ surgeries include arthroscopic removal of adhesions, coupled with insertion of anti-inflammatory agents, and open joint surgery, in which the joints are actually reconstructed.

## ORAL MANIFESTATIONS OF DEHYDRATION, ANEMIA, LUPUS, AND THROMBOCYTOPENIA

Oral health does not exist in isolation, and often can serve as an indicator of the patient's overall well-being. Many **systemic diseases present with oral manifestations** that the GCA must be familiar with:

- *Dehydration*: Prolonged dehydration results in decreased saliva production, dry mucus membranes, and dry tongue. Over time, these deficiencies can lead to an increase in dental caries. Any signs of dehydration that manifest orally should be investigated, as they may indicate chronic dehydration, which can be representative of a more serious underlying condition.
- *Anemia*: Iron-deficiency anemia manifests with pale gums and a smooth tongue (atrophic glossitis). The patient may also complain of a burning sensation of the tongue, gums and lips, a condition called angular cheilitis.
- *Systemic Lupus Erythematosus*: An autoimmune disease, SLE presents with oral manifestations in as high as 45% of its patients. These oral manifestations are most commonly oral lesions in the form of ulcers, erythematous, or hyperkeratosis.
- *Thrombocytopenia*: When thrombocytopenia is secondary to hematologic malignancy, it may first manifest in the oral cavity. Manifestations include petechiae or, when serious, hematomas or hemorrhagic bullae lesions. Minor trauma, such as probing the gum line, can also cause excessive bleeding in these patients.

## ORAL CONDITIONS CAUSED BY IMPROPER DIET

The most common **oral conditions caused by improper diet** are angular cheilitis and glossitis.

- *Angular cheilitis* is due to a shortage of Vitamin B complex. It presents as a lesion of both the mucous membranes and skin near the corner of the mouth, thus changing the vertical dimension of the face. Saliva accumulates at the corners and microorganisms proliferate there, particularly opportunistic infections like Candida albicans. The deficiency must be corrected and antifungal drugs are prescribed. Angular cheilitis can also develop if the person often licks the corners of his or her mouth, or drops vertical length in his or her face.
- Vitamin B complex deficiency is probably also the cause of *glossitis* or bald tongue, in which the tongue is inflamed and filiform papillae are lacking.

## ANOREXIA NERVOSA OR BULIMIA

**Anorexia nervosa** is an eating disorder characterized by unrealistic fears of consuming food and weight loss of at least 15%. **Bulimia** is an eating disorder distinguished by uncontrollable binge eating followed by self-induced vomiting. Eating disorder patients can die from electrolyte imbalance and heart attack. The appearance of the oral cavity changes due to vomiting accompanying bulimia: The lingual surfaces of the front teeth lose calcium; enamel wears away; occlusal faces of back teeth also erode. If the patient had restorative work, the fillings fail. Eating disordered patients tend to have many caries and enlarged parotid glands. Good oral hygiene is imperative, particularly after vomiting. Recommend toothpaste for sensitive teeth to eating disordered patients.

# Oral and Dental Anatomy, Physiology, and Development

## FEATURES OF THE TONGUE AND FLOOR OF MOUTH

The **dorsal (top) side of the tongue** has several types of papilla or projections in its anterior two-thirds, bearing the taste buds. The dorsal tongue has a groove, called the median sulcus, dividing the front portion in half, and another groove in the back, called the sulcus terminalis. Large circumvallated papillae are located in front of the sulcus terminalis. Hair-like protrusions, called filiform papillae, appear further forward. Redder, fungiform papillae appear near the front of the tongue. Tissue creases on the sides of the tongue are foliate papillae.

The **ventral (underside) of the tongue** has a central line of tissue, termed the lingual frenum, which continues into the floor of the mouth. There are lingual veins on its sides, and tissue creases, called fimbriated folds. At the point of attachment where the lingual frenum meets the floor of the mouth, there are tissue folds called sublingual caruncles. Sublingual folds branch from the caruncles. There is a sublingual sulcus close to the dental arch.

## MAJOR BLOOD VESSELS IN HEAD AND NECK

**Blood** is supplied to the head and neck from the subclavian arteries and the carotid arteries. The external carotid artery branches into the superior thyroid artery, lingual artery, facial artery, occipital artery, and posterior auricular arteries. The external carotid then divides into the maxillary and temporal arteries. The maxillary artery provides blood for the teeth, gums, jaws, cheek, nose, and eyelids. The temporal artery provides blood for the surface areas of face and scalp as well as the parotid glands. The internal carotid artery divides into the anterior and middle cerebral arteries, which supply blood to the brain. The ophthalmic artery is a branch of the internal carotid artery.

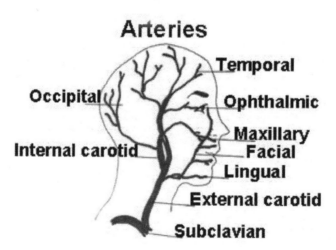

## BONE STRUCTURE

### MAXILLA AND PALATE

The **maxilla (upper jaw)** is the biggest facial bone, extending from the eye sockets and nasal cavities to form the roof of the oral cavity. The maxilla has two segments of bone, held together in the middle by the median suture. The maxilla develops from four bony outgrowths or processes: Frontal, zygomatic, alveolar, and palatine. The infraorbital foramen opens beneath the eye sockets. Sizeable maxillary sinuses open near the roots of the top molars, and there is a rounded area in the back, called the maxillary tuberosity. The palatine bones fuse at the midline along the palatine suture. The nasopalatine nerve connects to the palatine bones near the front at the incisive foramen. There is a horizontally located transverse palatine suture near the back of the hard palate.

Posterior to it on each side are three other openings, one greater palatine foramen, and two more diminutive, lesser palatine foramen.

## MANDIBLE

The only facial bone that can move is the **mandible (lower jaw).** It curves in front in the horizontal plane (following the dental arch), with vertical wings at the back, called rami. The rami are capped by two projections, the condyloid process in the back (which connects to the temporal bone to form the temporomandibular joint) and the sharper coronoid process, anterior to it. From the ramus area going forward, are the mandibular and mental foramen on the outside, and the lingual foramen on the tongue side. The latter has characteristic ridges. The front of the mandible is distinguished by a depression in its center, where the symphysis bones meet. The apex of the chin is the mental protuberance.

## CRANIAL AND FACIAL

**Cranial bones** enclose and protect the brain, and produce some red blood cells. There are two temporal bones at the lower sides and base of the skull and one frontal bone in the forehead. There are two parietal bones on the top and upper sides of the head. The occipital bone lies at the rear and base of the skull. The sphenoid bone is in front of the temporal area. The ethmoid bones create part of the nose, eye sockets, and floor of the cranium. Various processes and sinuses make the cranium light.

There are eight types of **facial bones**: A set of nasal bones constituting the bridge of the nose; one vomer bone inside, forming part of the nasal septum that separates the two nasal cavities; inferior nasal conchae inside the cavity that warm and filter air; two lacrimal bones that are part of the orbit of the eye; zygomatic bones create the cheeks and are also part of the maxilla or upper jaw; two maxilla; the palatine bones; and the mandible.

## TMJ

The **temporomandibular joint (TMJ)** is a junction formed by the glenoid fossa, and articular eminence of the temporal bone, and the condyloid process of the mandible. The temporal bones on either side of the face are cranial bones. The TMJ is immersed in synovial fluid, and its bones are enclosed by cartilage and supported by ligaments. The condyloid process or condyle is padded with fibrous connective tissue, called the articular disc or meniscus. When the mouth is closed, the meniscus is in close contact with the glenoid fossa of the temporal bone and the articular eminence further forward. The meniscus and glenoid are separated by cavities bathed in synovial fluid. As the mouth opens, a hinge motion develops, as the condyles and discs move forward. Then the condyles and discs move further forward, as the mouth opens more in a forward gliding joint movement. If the meniscus gets trapped or dislocated, TMJ disease manifests as a clicking noise and jaw pain.

## SALIVARY GLANDS

**Salivary glands** secrete saliva, a digestive fluid, into the oral cavity. Saliva moistens food and tissues in the oral space, facilitates chewing and ingestion, aids digestion of starches, and normalizes water balance. Saliva is a transparent liquid, normally of slightly alkaline pH. Saliva contains water, mucin protein, organic salts, and ptyalin enzyme. Saliva is secreted from three pairs of salivary glands and their adjoining ducts, which drain the saliva into the mouth. The parotid glands are located ahead of the ear; their parotid or Stensen's ducts empty into the area around the maxillary second molars. The submandibular glands are located in the rear of the mandible; their Warton's ducts drain into the sublingual caruncles. The sublingual glands are positioned on the floor of the mouth and can empty either right into the mouth via the ducts of Rivinus, or indirectly via the ducts of Bartholin into the sublingual caruncles.

## HEAD AND NECK MUSCLES

# Muscles

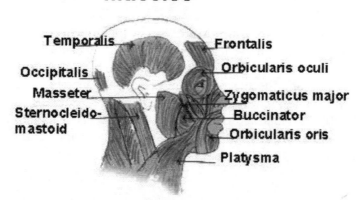

Temporalis
Occipitalis
Masseter
Sternocleido-
mastoid

Frontalis
Orbicularis oculi
Zygomaticus major
Buccinator
Orbicularis oris
Platysma

The epicranius covers the upper part of the skull and has two parts, frontalis and occipitalis, which are connected by a tendinous membrane. When the epicranius contracts, the forehead wrinkles and eyebrow raise. The orbicularis oculi surrounds the eye and allows it to open and close and controls the flow of tears. The orbicularis oris opens and closes the mouth. The buccinator muscle in the cheek helps to hold food next to the teeth for chewing. The zygomaticus major and minor allow the mouth to smile while the platysma helps lower the mandible and pulls the mouth down. The temporalis, which helps to raise the jaw, and the masseter, which also raises the jaw, are muscles of mastication along with underlying medial and lateral pterygoid muscles.

## CRANIAL AND FACIAL NERVES

Cranial and facial nerves are as follows:

1. Olfactory: Smell.
2. Optic: Vision.
3. Oculomotor
4. Trochlear: Eye muscle, upward movement.
5. Trigeminal: Chewing, sensory perception.
6. Abducens: Eye movement, lateral movement.
7. Facial: Expressions, tears, taste, saliva.
8. Vestibular: Balance and hearing.
9. Glossopharyngeal: Taste, mouth sensation.
10. Vagus: Swallowing, gag reflex.
11. Spinal accessory: Shoulder muscle movement.
12. Hypoglossal: Tongue

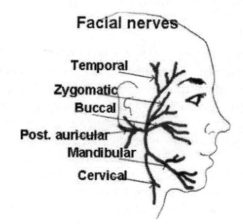

Facial nerves

Temporal
Zygomatic
Buccal
Post. auricular
Mandibular
Cervical

## LANDMARKS OF THE ORAL CAVITY

The **oral cavity** has a vestibule or mucobuccal fold, the pouch where the soft cheek and gums meet. Its continuous border is the vestibule fornix. There mucosa (moist linings) in the oral cavity are:

1. The *labial mucosa* on the inside of the lips.
2. The *buccal mucosa* on the interior of the cheeks.
3. The looser, redder *alveolar mucosa* encasing the alveolar bone, shoring up the teeth.

On the labial mucosa, near the corners of the mouth, are Fordyce's spots, minute yellow glands. The **buccal mucosa** has two characteristic features: An elevated white line where teeth meet, called the linea alba, and a piece of skin across from the maxillary second molar, known as the parotid papilla.

Another landmark is the **gingiva**, which are pink, fibrous gum tissue surrounding teeth. The oral cavity has two types of **frena** (restraining folds of tissue): The labial frena (the major ones between the central incisors in either jaw) and the buccal frena. Frenulum and frenum are both correct singulars of frena.

## LANDMARKS OF THE PALATE

The **palate** is the roof of the mouth, interior to the maxillary teeth. The front or hard palate is comprised of a bony plate, enveloped with pink keratinized tissue, and the back or soft palate, made of muscle.

| Hard Palate Landmarks | Soft Palate Landmarks |
|---|---|
| Incisive papilla (an elevated area behind the top central incisors), ridges that run either down the center toward the back. | Uvula, an outcrop of tissue at the entrance to the throat. |
| A single palatine raphe, running horizontally across the hard palate posterior to the incisive papilla, the palatine rugae. | Anterior tonsillar pillars that arch toward the tongue, and posterior tonsillar pillars extending behind the soft palate into the oropharynx. |
| Torus palatinus, a bony protuberance in the center of the palate. | Palatine tonsils located between the posterior pillars at the rear of the oral cavity in the fauces, the entrance to the pharynx. |

## TEETH
### DECIDUOUS AND PERMANENT DENTITION

There are **20 deciduous teeth** (10 in each arch, 5 in each quadrant). Starting at the midline and extending backwards, each quadrant contains: (1) central incisor (cutter); (2) lateral incisor (cutter); (3) canine or cuspid (tearer); (4) first molar (grinder); and (5) second molar (grinder).

**Thirty-two permanent teeth** (16 per arch, 8 per quadrant) function similarly to primary teeth. The permanent teeth in each quadrant, extending from the midline to the back of each arch, are: (1) central incisor; (2) lateral incisor; (3) canine; (4) first premolar; (5) second premolar (bicuspids choppers); (6) first molar; (7) second molar; and (8) third molar (grinder). The anterior teeth in the front of deciduous and permanent dentition are the central and lateral incisors and canines. Anterior teeth have single roots and a distinct incisal edge. Posterior teeth, behind the anterior teeth, have more than one root and cusp (grinding surface).

### ERUPTION AND EXFOLIATION SCHEDULE FOR PRIMARY DENTITION

Children's deciduous or **primary teeth begin erupting** around four to six months of age. Most children have a complete set of primary teeth by 32 months of age. The eruption schedule is similar for both the maxillary and mandibular arch. Central incisors erupt first, followed by the lateral incisors, the first molars, the canines, and lastly the second molars. Primary teeth are shed from the oral cavity or exfoliated in approximately the same order. Exfoliation generally starts at age 6 to 7 years, beginning with the central incisor. Exfoliation should be complete by 10 to 12 years of age. The canines and second molars shed last.

### ERUPTION SCHEDULE FOR PERMANENT DENTITION

From about age 6 to 12 years, a child has mixed dentition. **Permanent teeth begin to erupt** during this period before all primary teeth are shed. The permanent teeth that eventually replace the deciduous central incisors, lateral incisors, and canines are succedaneous (they succeed deciduous teeth). Molars are not succedaneous. The first molars are generally the first permanent teeth to come into both arches at about age 6 to 7 years, followed by the central incisors and lateral incisors. The other teeth may come in differently for the two arches. The second and third molars are the last teeth to appear (usually at ages 13 and 21, respectively).

## MORPHOLOGY OF PERMANENT POSTERIOR MAXILLARY TEETH

Morphology of permanent posterior maxillary teeth is described below:

- **Maxillary first and second premolars** (bicuspids) are posterior to the canines. Premolars have crowns with two cusps. The facial cusp is larger than the lingual cusp. The difference is more pronounced in the first premolar. Maxillary first premolars have two bifurcated roots, whereas maxillary second premolars have single roots.
- Proceeding posteriorly are the **maxillary first molars**, which are almost square and have five cusps: Mesio-buccal, disto-buccal, mesio-lingual, disto-lingual, and the cusp of Carabelli on the mesio-lingual cusp. There is a buccal groove between the mesio-buccal and disto-buccal cusps, and buccal and lingual pits, a central fossa, and oblique and transverse ridges. Maxillary first molars have trifurcated roots.
- **Maxillary second molars** are slightly smaller and have only four cusps (minus the cusp of Carabelli); they have trifurcated roots.
- **Maxillary third molars** are slighter than the second molars and have more grooves on the occlusal surface. Their root structure varies. Third molars may be absent or fail to erupt, requiring removal.

## MORPHOLOGY OF PERMANENT ANTERIOR MAXILLARY TEETH

The morphology of permanent anterior maxillary teeth is described below:

- **Maxillary incisors** have sharp incisal edges but no cusps. They have single roots up to twice the length of their crowns. The *maxillary central incisors* near the midline are slightly larger (both crown and root) than the adjacent maxillary lateral incisors. When central incisors initially erupt, they display three bumps on the incisal surface, called mamelons, which wear down to a flat edge. Incisors have imbrications, or faint overlapping lines and developmental depressions, on the labial surface near the gums. The labial surface of the crown is convex, while the lingual side is concave. Incisors are essential for producing certain speech sounds. *Maxillary lateral incisors* often vary from the expected.
- The **maxillary canines** (cuspids) have the longest roots in the maxillary arch, making them the most secure. The labial surface of the crown is convex with a vertical ridge. The incisal edge ends in a tip. The lingual side has two hollow fossae, separated by ridges. Canines contain more dentin (calcium-containing material) below the enamel, making canines darker than incisors.

## MORPHOLOGY OF PERMANENT POSTERIOR MANDIBULAR TEETH

The morphology of permanent posterior mandibular teeth is described below:

- The **mandibular first premolar** (bicuspid) has two cusps on the crown: A prominent buccal cusp and a smaller lingual cusp, with an occlusal groove between. There are mesial, distal, and transverse ridges. Mandibular first premolars have short, single, straight roots.
- The **mandibular second premolar** has up to three short lingual cusps and one buccal cusp. Three grooves and ridges are on the occlusal surface. Mandibular second premolars have one distally angled root.

- The **mandibular first molars** are the biggest teeth. They have five cusps, meeting on the occlusal face in a central fossa, with grooves in between cusps. The crown is concave on the mesial side but straight distally. This pattern reflects in the two root structures (mesial and distal). The mesial root has two separate pulp canals.
- The **mandibular second molar** is smaller than the first, with four cusps meeting on the occlusal surface, and buccal and lingual grooves that terminate in pits. Second molars usually have bifurcated roots.
- **Mandibular third molars** are smaller, with multiple roots and furrowed surfaces.

## MORPHOLOGY OF PERMANENT ANTERIOR MANDIBULAR TEETH

The morphology of permanent anterior mandibular teeth is described below:

- Contrary to dentition in the maxillary arch, the **mandibular central incisor** is smaller than the adjoining lateral incisor. Mandibular central incisors have single, very straight, pointed roots. The crowns are very slender and sharp at the edge. Initial mamelons wear off. Mandibular central incisors have convex labial and concave lingual surfaces and a cingulum. The only differences in the lateral incisors are larger crowns, with relatively smaller distal sides, and smaller single roots that may have concave surfaces.
- The **mandibular canines** (bicuspids) have single roots with deep depressions; they may be shorter than those of the maxillary canines in the upper arch. The crowns of mandibular canines have steeping sloping distal cusps and smaller mesial cusps.

## MORPHOLOGY OF DECIDUOUS MANDIBULAR TEETH

The morphology of deciduous mandibular teeth is described below:

- The **mandibular deciduous central incisor** is very similar to its permanent replacement, except its crown is wider and both lingual and labial surfaces are curved, while the sides are flat.
- **The mandibular deciduous lateral incisor**s are slightly longer and broader than the central incisors; they have a prominent cingulum, distal and mesial ridges, and a deeper fossa. Their roots bend distally at the bottom.
- **Mandibular deciduous canines** have smaller roots and less prominent crown ridges than their maxillary counterparts.
- **Mandibular deciduous incisors** and canines have single roots.
- The **mandibular deciduous first molars** have four cusps (mesio-buccal is the biggest), relatively long buccal facades, and bifurcated roots on the mesial and distal sides.
- **Mandibular deciduous second molars** look like permanent mandibular first molars, but are smaller. The mesio-buccal and disto-buccal cusps are about the same size. Mandibular deciduous second molars have two roots; the mesial root is bigger than the distal.

## MORPHOLOGY OF DECIDUOUS MAXILLARY TEETH

The morphology of deciduous maxillary teeth is described below:

- **Deciduous (primary) teeth** have relatively long roots compared to their crowns, more prominent cervical ridges, and are very white, due to thin enamel and dentin, but more pulp). Deciduous teeth are smaller than permanent teeth.
- **Maxillary deciduous central incisors** have distinct cervical lines, are wider than their height, have no mamelons, and their labial sides are convex.
- **Maxillary deciduous lateral incisors** are smaller, longer, and more curved than central incisors.

31

- **Maxillary deciduous canines (cuspids)** have pointed incisal rims, ridges on the mesial and distal sides, and prominent cingula. Maxillary deciduous cuspid roots are more elongated than the incisors. All of these anterior teeth have single roots.
- The **maxillary deciduous first molars** have four cusps, transverse and oblique ridges, and three roots. The mesio-lingual cusp is the most prominent.
- **Second molars** have four or five main cusps, and three widely separated roots.

## ANATOMICAL LANDMARKS OF TEETH

The following are anatomical landmarks of teeth:

- **Bifurcation or trifurcation:** 2 or 3 roots emerge from the tooth's main trunk. The dividing spot is the furcation.
- **Grooves or depressions**: 3 types: Buccal grooves, developmental grooves on the occlusal surface; and supplemental grooves emanating from the developmental type. Fissures are imperfectly united developmental grooves. Pits are areas where fissures meet.
- **Ridges:** Elevated sections of enamel. 4 types: marginal, oblique, transverse and triangular. Only marginal ridges are found on anterior teeth. All 4 types are observed on molars.
- **Fossa:** Relatively superficial rounded or angular depressions
- **Apex**: At or near the terminus of the root; the apical foramen is an opening at the apex through which nerves and blood vessels come into the tooth.
- **Cusp:** Mounds on the crown; most molars have multiple cusps. First molars may also have a fifth cusp on the mesial lingual surface, known as the Cusp of Carabelli. Lobes are united partitions that form teeth (usually equivalent to cusps for molars).
- **Cingulum**: Convex space on lingual surface of front teeth.
- **Mamelons**: 3 protuberances on incisal edge of new central incisors.

## DENTAL ARCHES AND QUADRANTS

Dentition is the normal arrangement of teeth in the mouth. Teeth grow in one of two **dental arches**. Teeth set into the maxilla (upper jawbone) comprise the maxillary arch, which is affixed to the skull and has no flexible sideways movement. Teeth set in the mandible (lower jawbone) comprise the mandibular arch, which is flexible and can move sideways and up and down. Adjoining teeth that are correctly positioned touch each other. Maxillary arch teeth contact and slightly overlap those in the mandibular arch when the patient closes his or her mouth.

**Dental quadrants** are areas of dentition defined by the arch they are in (to the right or left side of the midline of the face). Thus, there are four dental quadrants: Maxillary right quadrant, maxillary left quadrant, mandibular right quadrant and mandibular left quadrant. The primary or deciduous teeth grown initially by children number 20, so there are 5 teeth in each quadrant. There are 32 permanent teeth developed in adolescence, with 8 in each quadrant.

# Charting

## Descriptive Charting Terms

Some **basic charting terms** that are **descriptive** include:

- *Abscess* - A deep, limited, infected pocket filled with pus.
- *Diastema* - The gap between two teeth, usually used to describe that between maxillary central incisors.
- *Drifting* - Movement of tooth position to occupy spaces formed by removal of another, also called over eruption.
- *Incipient* - Areas of developing decay where enamel is still intact, appearance is chalky due to initiation of decalcification.
- *Mobility* - Movement of a tooth within the socket quantified in millimeters; generally, results from trauma or periodontal disease.
- *Periodontal pocket* - Excessive space (more than 3 mm) in a gum sulcus, due to periodontal disease.
- *Overhang* - Presence of too much restorative material.

## Charting Symbols

The following are some typical charting symbols for caries, restorations, crowns, and prosthetic devices:

- Red indicates **caries** that have not yet been restored; blue indicates caries that were restored. Either fill in the affected surface on the chart, or encircle it with the appropriate color.
- Chart **amalgam restorations** by both outlining and filling in. Show composites with outlining only.
- Indicate **recurrent decay** of previously restored teeth by outlining the existing restoration in red.
- For **enamel sealants** that have been used to deter decay, place an "S" over the area.
- **Temporary restorations** are indicated with blue circles.
- For **crowns**, draw diagonal lines across the whole area involved if gold, or encircle if porcelain.
- For **fixed bridges**, draw an "X" through the root(s) of missing teeth; the area for the bridge is either outlined (porcelain) or indicated by diagonal lines (gold).
- Show a **Maryland bridge**, which has wings on the pontic, with curves.
- Indicate **veneers** by outlining.
- For **dentures**, place "X"s over all involved root areas, and show the corresponding crown areas by either a large circle (full) or dotted lines (partial).

The following are some typical charting symbols for missing, drifting, impacted, or to be extracted teeth, and other anomalies:

- Indicate **future dental work** in red on a chart.
- Indicate completed dental work in blue.
- Place an "X" through **missing teeth** on the chart. If all the teeth in an arch are missing, encircle and place an "X" over it.
- Draw supernumerary (extra) teeth on the chart.
- Show **drifting or overerupted teeth** by drawing arrows in the direction of the drift.

- Circle impacted or unerupted teeth.
- Place a red slash through **teeth requiring extraction**.
- Indicate **diastema** with two vertical lines at the gap.
- Show **tooth rotation** with a directional arrow on the side.
- Indicate **mobility** with two small lines.
- Draw jagged lines to indicate **tooth or root fracture**.
- If a tooth needs a **root canal**, draw vertical red lines through it. If the root canal procedure has already been performed, draw blue vertical lines through it.
- Show **gingival recession** or furcation involvement with wavy lines and dots.
- A small red circle drawn near the root indicates an **abscess**.
- Arrows between roots indicate **periodontal pockets**.

## TOOTH DIAGRAMS AND CODING SYSTEMS

**Tooth diagrams** are either anatomic or geometric. An anatomic diagram has pictures that look like real teeth, including the roots. A geometric diagram uses divided circles to represent each tooth. The circle's divisions signify different tooth surfaces. Each chart has positions for all 16 upper and 16 lower teeth.

Several **different numbering systems** may be used. The most common in the USA is the Universal/National System. Other countries use the International Standards Organization System more often. The teeth are shown as if one is looking into the patient's mouth. Indicate completed dental treatments in either blue or black on the chart. Note newly detected or incomplete treatments in red. Use Black's classification system to mark cavities (caries) on the diagram as Classes I to VI. Dental offices may use a variety of symbols or short forms to describe conditions or materials used in the patient's mouth. Ask the office manager for a copy of acceptable abbreviations to avoid confusion.

## UNIVERSAL/NATIONAL SYSTEM OF NUMBERING TEETH

The **Universal/National System** is sanctioned by the American Dental Association and is the most common system used to number teeth in the United States. Children's primary teeth are lettered from A to J in the maxilla (upper jaw) from the right second molar to the left second molar. Children's mandibular (lower jaw) teeth are lettered from K to T starting with the left second molar and ending with the right second molar. Adults' permanent teeth are designated numbers from 1 to 32. Number 1 starts on the maxilla at the upper right third molar, and proceeds consecutively along the top to tooth #16 on the upper left third molar. Numbering of the lower teeth starts on the mandible at the left third molar as tooth #17 and ends at tooth #32 or the lower-right third molar.

## ALTERNATIVE TOOTH NUMBERING SYSTEMS

Most foreign countries use the **International Standards Organization System/Federation Dentaire Internationale (ISO/FDI).** Two digits identify each tooth: The first is the quadrant and the second is the tooth. Start numbering in the center of the mouth for adults and children. The first digit 1 is the adult's right maxillary quadrant; 2 is left maxillary; 3 is left mandibular; and 4 is right mandibular. The second digit for permanent teeth in each adult quadrant runs from 1 to 8, starting at the incisors. Number children's quadrants from 5 to 8 for primary teeth. Children's second digits extend from 1 to 5 because they have fewer teeth. Pronounce digits separately, e.g., "One one", rather than "Eleven."

The UK uses **Palmer Notation (Military System).** Bracket symbols indicate the quadrant. The digit, representing the tooth, proceeds from the center. Number permanent teeth from 1 to 8. Number primary teeth from A to E.

## PALMER NOTATION METHOD

**Palmer Notation Method** (Adults)

- In this system, the mouth is divided into four sections called quadrants. The numbers 1 through 8 and a unique symbol are used to identify the teeth in each quadrant. The numbering runs from the center of the mouth to the back.
- In the upper right section of the mouth, for example, tooth number 1 is the incisor (flat, front tooth) just to the right of the center of the mouth. The numbers continue to the right and back to tooth number 8, which is the wisdom tooth (third molar.)
- The numbers sit inside an L-shaped symbol used to identify the quadrant. The "L" is right side up for the teeth in the upper right. The teeth in the upper left use a backward "L." For the bottom quadrants, the "L" is upside-down. The quadrants may also be identified by letters, such as "UR" or "URQ" for the upper right quadrant.

## DIVISIONS AND SURFACES OF TEETH

Each tooth has:

- A **crown** enclosed by enamel.
- A **root** faced with a thin layer of bony tissue called cementum.
- A **cervical line** (the cementoenamel junction) dividing the two.

Anatomical surfaces describe the actual covering material of crowns and roots. Clinical surfaces refer to the visible portion of the crown and root.

- **Anterior teeth** have 5 crown surfaces: (1) mesial, facing the midline; (2) distal, facing away from the midline; (3) labial, exterior opposite the lips; (4) lingual or palatal, interior facing the tongue; and (5) incisal or cutting edge.
- **Posterior teeth** also have five coronal surfaces: (1) mesial; (2) distal; (3) lingual; (4) buccal, exterior toward the cheek; and (5) occlusal, the top chewing surface.

Another term for labial or buccal surfaces is facial. Surfaces can be convex (curving outward), or concave (curving inward), or flat. Any combination of surfaces can be found on the same tooth.

### CHARTING SURFACES INVOLVED WITH CAVITIES

**Cavities** are charted in terms of whether they involve one, two, three, or more surfaces that have been or need to be restored. A simple cavity restoration involves only a single surface. Simple cavity restorations are described by a letter standing for the surface involved: I (incisal); M (mesial); D (distal); B (buccal); O (occlusal) or F (facial). Compound or two-surface restorations use a combination of two letters that illustrate the two facades involved. Thus, typical compound cavity restorations are described as: OB (occlusobuccal); MO (mesio-occlusal); MI (mesio-incisal); DO (disto-occlusal); DI (disto-incisal); DL (disto-lingual); or LI (lingual-incisal). Complex cavity restorations involve at least three surfaces and the abbreviations for them incorporate all facades involved, for example MOD for mesio-occluso-distal.

### DESCRIPTIVE TERMS FOR RELATIONSHIPS EXPRESSED IN CAVITY PREPARATIONS

**Cavity preparation** creates walls, lines and angles within the tooth. Walls are any side or floor of the preparation. They are described in terms of the nearest tooth surface, for example distal, buccal, pulpal (over the pulp), axial (parallel to the tooth's long axis), or gingival (perpendicular to the long axis). Lines are created when two surfaces converge. Preparation is described in terms of the line angles that result, for example, the buccopulpal line angle or mesiobuccal line angle. When three surfaces converge, they form point angles, for example, the mesiobuccopulpal point angle or distobuccopulpal point angle. Another angle is the cavosurface margin, which is the angle between the preparation and untouched tooth surface; it is important to seal these surfaces. In any cavity preparation, there are numerous line and point angles. Cavities are described in terms of depth. An ideal depth is shallow enough to retain the restorative material, a moderate depth is a slightly deeper one that does not invade the pulp, and a very deep preparation very nearly or actually exposes pulp.

## CLASSIFICATIONS OF DENTAL CARIES AND APPROPRIATE DENTAL MATERIALS

Dental caries (cavities) are **classified** from Class I to Class VI based on the teeth and surfaces they are formed in. Classes I to V were described by a pioneer in the field of dentistry, G. V. Black, and Class VI was included later. They are:

- *Class I* - Developmental caries in pits and fissures, including occlusal surfaces of back teeth, buccal or lingual pits on molars, and lingual pits on maxillary incisors. Restore with tooth-colored composite resins.
- *Class II* - Cavities on proximal surfaces of premolars or molars. Restore with tooth-colored resins, silver amalgam, gold or porcelain.
- *Class III* - Cavities on interproximal surfaces of incisors or canines. Restore with composite resins.
- *Class IV* - Similar to Class III except incisal edge is also involved. Restored with composites, and if considerably decayed, porcelain crowns.
- *Class V* - Caries only near the gum line on either facial or lingual surface. Restore with composites for front teeth and silver amalgam for posterior teeth
- *Class VI* - Cavities on occlusal or incisal surfaces formed by erosion. Various restoration materials are appropriate.

## UPDATED CLASSIFICATION SCHEME FOR PERIODONTITIS

In 2018, the American Academy of Periodontology and the European Federation of Periodontology agreed to adopt an **updated classification system for periodontitis** that reflects the complexity of the disease. These changes were agreed upon at the 2017 World Workshop on the Classification of Periodontal and Peri-Implant Disease and Conditions. The updated classification system incorporates a staging and grading process that reflections the multidimensional view of periodontitis.

The **staging process** examines the severity (combining an assessment of interdental CAL, radiographic bone loss and tooth loss due to periodontitis), complexity (maximum probing depth and bone loss) and extent/distribution of the disease (described as either local, generalized or molar/incisor pattern). A stage (I-IV) is the applied to the disease based on these factors. This stage applies to the full mouth rather than just one region or zone of the mouth. The condition is then **graded** based on progression (indirect or direct evidence), which is influenced by grade modifiers (risk factors such as smoking or diabetes). Grading is as follows: Grade A (slow rate of progression), Grade B (moderate rate of progression), and Grade C (rapid rate of progression).

This new system is meant to specify the diagnosis and guide treatment of the disease.

## DENTAL CHARTING OF PERIODONTAL CONDITIONS OR PRECURSORS

Excessive **dental plaque** leads to periodontal disease. Indicate plaque on the chart by a squiggly line above the tooth. Indicate periodontal pockets with an arrow and number indicating depths. A full periodontal chart enumerates the periodontal pocket depth for each tooth on both the facial and lingual sides. The dentist or hygienist "walks" the probe around the tooth and takes six distinct sulcal measurements (mesio-buccal, midbuccal, distobuccal, distolingual, mid-lingual, and mesio-lingual). Classify **tooth mobility** as normal (0), slight (1), moderate (2) or severe (3). Note areas of exudate or pus. Show gingival recession by drawing a dotted or colored line along the gum line, to illustrate root exposure. Note furcation involvement for the molars only.

## CHARTING TERMS THAT REFER TO COMPLETED OR SUGGESTED DENTAL WORK

Basic charting terms referring to **completed or suggested dental work** include:

- *Bridge* - A prosthesis that replaces missing teeth, held in place on attaching sides (abutments), or sometimes just one side (a cantilever bridge). The middle area is termed the pontic.
- *Crown* – Permanent, custom-made or manufactured temporary tooth covers. Crowns are available in a variety of materials and combinations, including gold, porcelain, stainless steel, and plastic. A crown covers either the full tooth or ¾ of the tooth.
- *Denture* - A complete (full arch) or partial set of artificial teeth attached to a plate.
- *Restoration* - Materials used to fill caries or replace missing tooth structure, including silver amalgams, composite resins, and gold.
- *Root canal* - A procedure in which the dentist removes the tooth pulp and replaces it with a filling material.
- *Sealant* – A resin used to seal pits and fissures in the tooth enamel to deter decay.
- *Veneer* – A thin material bonded only to the facial aspect of the tooth, usually for cosmetic improvement.

## DOCUMENTATION

**Documentation** must always be done during patient care or immediately afterward to ensure that no important information is forgotten or overlooked. The certified dental assistant should make objective observations as opposed to subjective:

- *Subjective*: Patient states he is "in severe pain from toothache."
- *Objective*: Patient moaning and holding right side of face.

All encounters (in-person, telephone, email) must be documented. Patient's acceptance of treatment should be documented, explaining the treatment and the patient response. Compliance or lack of compliance with the treatment regimen must be documented at each visit and contact. When appropriate, a consent form must be signed and witnessed and entered into the permanent record. If a patient refuses treatment or refuses to follow through with advice, this information must be documented along with the patient's reason and the patient asked to sign the statement as well if utilizing a paper record. In some cases, the patient may be asked to sign a "Refusal of Medical Advice" document, which is stored in the permanent record.

# Diagnostic Aids

## X-Ray

**Dental x-rays** enable the dentist to more thoroughly evaluate dental health. These images use low levels of radiation to produce images of the inside of the teeth and gums. Different types of dental x-rays can identify different types of dental problems:

- *Bitewing x-rays* are images of the upper and lower teeth that identify cavities between the teeth, missing fillings, damaged crowns, or problems with the roots of the teeth.
- *Periapical x-rays* are images of the upper and lower teeth that are used for identifying problems in the roots of the teeth or in the surrounding bony tissue of the jaw.
- *Occlusal x-rays* are images of the upper and lower teeth. These images are larger and enable the dentist to visualize development and placement of the teeth.
- *Extraoral x-rays* are not used to identify cavities or other problems within the teeth. These images are used to visualize the jaws and skull surrounding the teeth to evaluate tooth placement, tooth impactions, and the bony development of the jaws in relation to the teeth.

## Photographs

**Intraoral and extraoral photographs** have several uses in dental practice.

- Obtaining photographs upon the initial assessment of a patient provides the baseline at which a patient started before undergoing any dental treatments of procedures. These should be stored in the patient's chart and can be used to compare the appearance of dental structures before and after undergoing dental work.
- Dental photographs are useful for patient education purposes to clearly show specific dental problems that are identified. Images of corrected dental problems can be used to compare a patient's current dental health to expected outcomes following a specific procedure.
- Changes in dental hygiene can be visualized with dental photographs. Showing the patient images of their gum disease before and after treatment is performed can help them to visualize the benefits of treatments and preventive measures that have been implemented.
- A library of images can be used for marketing purposes for the practice to show before and after pictures of dental work that has been completed. These can show the success the dentist has in treating various types of dental disease.

## Intraoral vs. Extraoral Photographs

**Intraoral photographs** enable the dentist to visualize areas of the oral cavity that are not easily visualized with the naked eye. Digital photographs can allow the dentist to enlarge images of the teeth to closely examine the condition of the tooth surface and enamel. Images of the surrounding gums and soft tissue can be enlarged to more closely examine any sites of potential dental disease. Enlarging the intraoral images enables the dentist to closely examine any cracks or imperfections in the surface of the tooth or early stages of gum disease or irritation that would not otherwise be seen until the condition progresses. These images can also be shared with patients so they can clearly see any potential problems within the mouth.

**Extraoral photographs** are taken to capture the alignment of the mouth and jaw as they relate to all of the facial structures. Images of the patient's face while it is at rest and while smiling are helpful for viewing before and after images to show improvement after orthodontic work or after treatments to help realign the jaws.

# Medical Conditions and Emergencies

## EMERGENCY PREPAREDNESS PROCEDURES

The **role of each person in the dental office during an emergency** should be clearly identified in the job description and rehearsed. For example:

- The *front desk receptionist* phones EMS, notifies the dentist, directs traffic, and reschedules patients
- The *assistant* obtains the crash cart, provides first aid, and assists the dentist with life support
- The *hygienist* provides first aid, and contacts the patient's next-of-kin and physician
- The *dentist* leads two-person CPR and administers resuscitation drugs

Staff must cross train in various roles during routine practice drills, in case of absences or multiple casualties. Clearly post these emergency telephone numbers at Reception and in each treatment room: Emergency medical services (EMS); fire department; police; nearest hospital Emergency Room; oral surgeon; nearby doctor; Public Health; morgue. The universal emergency number is 911, except in some rural areas.

## DENTAL OFFICE EMERGENCY KIT

A **dental office emergency kit** should be maintained and updated in every dental office. Each treatment room should have a self-contained oxygen inhalation unit (with a green oxygen tank) or a wall-piped system for nitrous oxide gas and oxygen. Test the oxygen tank(s) weekly. The dental office emergency kit should contain: Plastic or metal airways; tracheotomy needles; masks for cardiopulmonary resuscitation; tourniquets; sterile syringes; antihistamines to counteract allergic reactions; an Epi-pen (epinephrine); vasodilators like nitroglycerin to increase blood flow and treat high blood pressure (hypertension); a vasopressor, like Wyamine, to treat low blood pressure (hypotension); anti-convulsants, like Diazepam; atropine to block the vagal nerve and increase the pulse rate; and analgesics (pain relievers). Check the medications monthly for expiration dates. Replace when needed.

## AMBU-BAG

An **Ambu-bag** is the proprietary name for a portable manual resuscitator or bag-valve-mask (BVM) device. Anytime a patient has an emergency involving respiratory failure or arrest, it is essential to deliver positive pressure oxygen to increase the relative amount of oxygen in the lungs, blood, and ultimately the brain. The preferred method is delivery of oxygen from a pressurized oxygen tank via a hose and mask. Emergencies occurring where an oxygen tank is unavailable can be addressed with an Ambu-bag, which has a self-inflating bag that fills up with air (and sometimes additional oxygen attached to a flexible mask), and seals to the patient's face. Positive pressure ventilation is delivered when the rescuer compresses the valve joining the bag and mask. Another portable method of resuscitation is a pocket mask, where the rescuer inflates the patient's lungs using exhaled air.

## MAGILL INTUBATION FORCEPS

Small dental tools and debris may dislodge in the patient's mouth during a procedure, causing obstruction. Intubation means placement of a tube into the airway to supply oxygen when the patient is unable to breathe independently due to obstruction. The dentist passes a long, curved **Magill intubation forceps** into the windpipe for endotracheal intubation and retrieval of objects obstructing the airway that are still visible. The assistant must be present to suction the mouth. Do not allow the patient to sit up during retrieval, as movement can result in further injury and force the object farther down the throat. If only one professional is present, or if the airway is partially obstructed, then tell the patient to bend his or her head down over the side of the chair and try to cough it free. Call 911. If full obstruction occurs, perform the Heimlich maneuver.

## ABCs of Cardiopulmonary Resuscitation

**Cardiopulmonary resuscitation (CPR)** is an emergency technique to revive a person whose heart has stopped beating. The process of CPR follows an ABC (and often D) pattern:

- "A" represents the *airway*, which must be first be opened up to allow air flow.
- "B" signifies *breathing*, which the rescuer must observe and work to re-establish if the patient is not breathing using rescue breathing or bag-mask ventilation.
- "C" stands for *circulation*, which the rescuer must check using the carotid pulse; if there is no pulse, then chest compressions interspersed with slow breaths are used to re-establish a pulse. Chest compressions should be at a rate of 100-120 compressions per minute at a depth of about 2 inches in adults.
- "D" refers to *defibrillation* using an automated external defibrillator (AED) unit, if available. Follow the AED's automated prompts to safely utilize this intervention.

Dental assistants are legally required to recertify in CPR with the American Red Cross or the American Heart Association every two years at the Healthcare Provider Level.

## CPR for Adult Victim with Single Rescuer

The dental assistant or dentist performs **CPR** on patients with cardiac arrest. The patient must be unresponsive, with no pulse or breathing.

1. Call Emergency Medical Services (911) before beginning.
2. Don gloves, if possible.
3. Place the patient supine on the floor.
4. Look, listen, and feel for the patient's pulse breathing. If there is no breathing, open the patient's airway by inclining the head back and raising the chin.
5. Place a resuscitation mouthpiece patient's mouth. Pinch the nose closed. Inflate the lungs with two breaths. Observe the chest's rise and fall.
6. Check the carotid pulse for about 10 seconds. If no pulse is present, kneel beside the patient.
7. Landmark the xiphoid process.
8. Place the palms over the breastbone. Compress 15 times, followed by two breaths.
9. After four cycles, check the carotid pulse again.
10. Continue until the patient breathes or relieved by a rescuer with higher training.
11. Discard the mouthpiece.
12. Document CPR in the patient's chart.

## AED Unit

An **automated external defibrillator (AED)** can revive a person in cardiac arrest if it is applied within four minutes and damage is not extensive. Continue CPR until the unit is charged. The patient must be on a flat, dry surface. Connect the electrodes of the AED to the patient, as illustrated on the unit. Press the "analyze" button first for a readout, to ensure the unit is ready and electroshock is appropriate. Announce, "Stay clear of the patient." Restart CPR if defibrillation is contraindicated. The unit indicates by tone or light that it is ready to shock the patient. Make sure that everyone is clear of the patient, and press the appropriate "shock" button on the AED. The AED display shows when defibrillation occurs. Resume CPR immediately after the shock is administered. Check the pulse after the third shock, or follow the AED's instructions if a pulse is detected. If there is a pulse, check the airway, breathing circulation and move the patient into recovery position. If there is no pulse, perform CPR for one minute before rechecking the pulse. If there is still no pulse, defibrillate again. Press the analysis button. Nine defibrillations can be performed. The unit indicates when to stop defibrillation.

## RESCUE BREATHING

**Rescue breathing** in emergency situations may be performed by the dental assistant, hygienist, nurse, or dentist if the patient is orally unresponsive. Call Emergency Medical Services (911) before beginning. Gloves are suggested but not required. If the patient is not breathing, tilt the head back and raise the chin to open the airway. Look, listen and feel for breathing. If there is none, insert a resuscitation mouthpiece into the patient's mouth. Pinch the nose closed. Provide two breaths to make the patient's chest rise. If it does not rise, assess the airway. If there is a visible source of obstruction, remove it, but do not do a blind sweep, as this risks pushing an object further into the airway. Check the carotid pulse in the neck, using the middle and forefingers. Perform rescue breathing while there is still a pulse, one slow breath every five seconds for a minute, followed by a pulse check. Repeat the sequence until breathing is re-established or a more qualified person takes over. If the pulse stops, begin CPR. When the incident concludes, throw the mouthpiece into a biohazard container. Document the incident.

## OXYGEN ADMINISTRATION

The dental assistant can **administer oxygen** in emergency situations. A crash cart contains a green oxygen tank, masks, airways, a defibrillator, and resuscitation drugs. One crash cart should be available per floor; remember where it is located. Tell the receptionist to call an ambulance (911) and notify the dentist. Place the patient in the supine position, lying on their back. If in true distress, place the patient on the floor if possible, as this position is safest and most effective for CPR. Position the oxygen mask over the patient's nose and mouth, with tubing to the side. Fasten the mask firmly. Administer oxygen without delay, at a rate of between 2 and 4 liters a minute. If the patient is still conscious, help reassure the patient and encourage them to take slow deep breaths. Try to calm and comfort the patient. Cover the patient with a blanket to help prevent shock. The dentist or registered nurse intubates the unconscious patient and administers resuscitation drugs.

## ALLERGIC REACTION

An **allergic reaction** is a response to exposure to a foreign agent (antigen). The patient's immune system develops antibodies to the antigen. Subsequent exposures to the antigen set off an allergic or hypersensitivity response, in which large amounts of histamine and other chemicals are released. Mild allergic reactions include skin reddening (erythema) and hives (urticaria). Remove the irritant and dispense antihistamines. Chronic allergy produces eczema. Asthma is a moderate allergic response in the airways. Anaphylactic shock is a possibly fatal allergic reaction. Allergens in the bloodstream stimulate histamine release, causing an immediate depression in blood pressure, airway constriction, swelling of the throat and tongue, and stomach pain. Give epinephrine immediately with an Epi-pen in the thigh muscle. Call 911. Administer oxygen, if required. The patient needs hospital follow-up within 20 minutes.

## ASTHMA

**Asthma** is a respiratory disease. It is often triggered by allergies or exposure to cold air, and is characterized by breathlessness and wheezing upon expiration. Asthma attacks are most likely to occur in the morning. A patient with asthma has narrowed bronchioles (small airways) in the lung. During exhalation, the lung collapses and bronchiole narrowing is exacerbated further, making it increasingly difficult to breathe. Administer antihistamines, such as albuterol, using an inhaler. The patient exhales first, and then inhales the bronchodilator drug through the device's mouthpiece, while depressing the canister portion. Bronchodilators expand the bronchioles to enhance airflow. Usually, two inhalations of bronchodilator will allay an attack and improve breathing in about 15 minutes. If not, dispense oxygen and call Emergency Services (911). Status asthmaticus is prolonged bronchial spasms, which can be fatal.

## BLOOD AND BLOOD DYSCRASIAS

Blood transports nutrients, antibodies, drugs, and diseases throughout the body. Blood helps to regulate body temperature and pH. Antibodies and white cells (leukocytes) in blood protect against infection. Clotting factors and calcium in blood protect against injury. Blood is 55% liquid plasma and 45% formed elements. The **three types of blood corpuscles** are:

- *Erythrocytes* (red cells or RBCs) containing the oxygen carrier protein hemoglobin
- *Leukocytes* (white cells or WBCs) that fight disease
- *Thrombocytes* (platelets) involved with blood clotting

People with **blood dyscrasias** have misshapen corpuscles or imbalanced blood elements. Dental assistants must beware of hemophilia, a hereditary lack of clotting Factor VIII that causes the male patient to bleed uncontrollably with the slightest injury. Leukemia, a progressive blood cancer in which abnormal leukocytes grow uncontrollably, causes the lymph nodes to swell. Hence, the dentist may be the first practitioner to diagnose leukemia.

## MALIGNANT ORAL TUMORS

Squamous cell and basal cell carcinomas are **malignant tumors**. Squamous epithelial cell carcinoma is the predominant oral cancer. It metastasizes (spreads through the lymph nodes) quickly. Predisposing factors include tobacco use, alcohol use, and exposure to sunlight. Squamous cell carcinomas initially look like white plaques that later ulcerate. Basal cell carcinoma is the chief form of skin cancer, again caused primarily by sunlight exposure. Fortunately, basal cell carcinoma rarely metastasizes and lesions can be surgically removed. Red patches in the oral cavity that are not due to inflammation are erythroplakia. Red patches are usually found on the floor of the mouth, the soft palate, or retro molar pad. They are associated with chronic tobacco or alcohol use, and they are almost without exception malignant or premalignant. Early erythroplakia is treated surgically. Late stage erythroplakia receives radiation and chemotherapy. Leukoplakia is unidentifiable white, tough, hyperkeratinized patches in the mucosa that cannot be wiped off, and are potentially malignant.

## WARNING SIGNALS OF ORAL CANCER

**Suspect oral cancer (malignancy)** if the patient displays any of the following warning signals:

- A sore in the oral cavity that does not resolve within about a month.
- Protracted mouth dryness.
- Lumps or areas of swelling in the region, including lips, oral cavity, or neck.
- White or coarse lesions on the lips or in the oral cavity.
- Numbness.
- Tenderness.
- Burning sensations in or anywhere near the oral cavity.
- Unexplained, recurrent bleeding in one part of the mouth.
- Difficulty speaking.
- Difficulty chewing or swallowing (dysphagia).
- Report findings to the dentist immediately. The dentist must refer the patient to an M.D. for follow-up.

## EPILEPTIC SEIZURE

**Epilepsy** is a brain disorder, in which disorganized electrical impulses hop the hemispheres in a "storm." Epilepsy can occur through head injuries, drug withdrawal, high fever, and metabolic imbalances. Tonic/clonic seizures (formerly called grand mal) are convulsions. The patient jerks and twitches, becomes unconscious for up to 5 minutes, followed by incontinence and exhaustion. Prolonged convulsions are status epilepticus, which is potentially fatal. Call EMS in the case of status epilepticus. Absence seizures (formerly called petit mal) are brief periods of blank staring and withdrawal. During partial seizures, an epileptic either retains consciousness (simple) or loses consciousness (complex). Both forms manifest as involuntary twitching; the main difference is recall ability. Absence and partial seizure do not require treatment. Stop the procedure. Remove all instruments from the mouth. After the seizure, place the patient on the right side with the airway open.

## HYPOGLYCEMIA

**Hypoglycemia** is too low a concentration of blood glucose (less than 70 mg/dl). It is caused by fasting, overexertion, stress, and drug reactions. Its symptoms are irritability nervousness, shaking, weakness, cold sweats, and hunger. Stop the procedure. Give 8 ounces of orange juice, or a glucose drink, or 6 glucose tablets, or 10 Lifesavers candies immediately. A delay may cause the patient to become unresponsive and require glucagon injections, or hospital treatment for acidosis. If the patient loses consciousness, call EMS (911) and apply a tablespoon of sugar to the buccal mucosa. Excess amounts of insulin can produce severe hypoglycemia and a critical drop in blood sugar, called insulin shock; in this case, intravenous glucose is indicated.

## TYPE I AND TYPE II DIABETES MELLITUS

**Type I (juvenile) diabetes mellitus** is a hereditary condition in which beta cells in the pancreas cannot produce insulin, a hormone that regulates glucose levels in the blood. Type I diabetics are insulin-dependent, meaning they must receive frequent injections of insulin to regulate blood sugar levels. Too much glucose in the blood is hyperglycemia, causing thirst, frequent urination, confusion, nausea, vomiting, abdominal pain, drunken behavior, and snoring. Too little glucose is hypoglycemia, with irritability, shaking, sweating, and loss of consciousness. Stop the procedure. Give the Type I diabetic his or her insulin pen or portable pump to prevent diabetic acidosis and possible coma. Type II diabetes mellitus patients have decreased sensitivity to insulin, with high blood glucose, obesity, and fatigue. Type II diabetes is probably not hereditary and tends to occur in adults. Type II diabetics can control their condition through diet and oral hypoglycemics. All diabetics have difficulty healing wounds.

> **Review Video: Diabetes Mellitus: Diet, Exercise, & Medications**
> Visit mometrix.com/academy and enter code: 774388

## ANGINA PECTORIS

**Angina pectoris** is chest pain. It indicates arterial damage and may lead to a heart attack if left untreated. Arteriosclerosis is hardening and narrowing of the arteries from plaque buildup, resulting in decreased blood flow to the heart. The patient may complain of chest pressure, or tightening, or a heavy weight behind the sternum. Pain may radiate up the neck or down the arms. If an episode of angina pectoris occurs in the dental office, stop the procedure. Check for increased blood pressure and pulse rate. Allow the patient to take sublingual nitroglycerin pills or spray to open up the coronary arteries and supply the heart with more oxygenated blood. Give the patient oxygen by mask. The patient can take up to three doses of nitroglycerin, spaced 3 to 5 minutes apart, before considering it a myocardial infarction (heart attack) and calling 911.

## Myocardial Infarction

A **myocardial infarction (MI)** or heart attack is an event in which a portion of heart tissue dies rapidly (necrosis), due to severe blockage or narrowing of the coronary arteries. The symptoms of MI are angina pectoris, ashen skin color, blue lips and ear lobes, and copious sweating. Unlike angina pectoris, chest pain from myocardial infarction cannot be assuaged with nitroglycerin administration. If an MI occurs in the dental office, terminate the procedure. Call 911. Reposition the patient with his or her head slightly raised. Administer oxygen and nitroglycerine. Alleviate the patient's stress.

MI is more prevalent in males, smokers, people older than 40, and diabetics. Heart disease can be controlled somewhat through diet, exercise, and lowering stress and blood pressure.

## Congestive Heart Failure

**Congestive heart failure (CHF)** is eventually terminal. The heart is unable to pump sufficient blood to meet the needs of all organs. CHF affects five million people in the USA. Older adults are most at risk. Causes of CHF include previous heart attack, hypertension, coronary artery disease, cardiomyopathy, congenital heart defects, valvular disease, cardiotoxic drugs, myocarditis and endocarditis. Signs and symptoms are shortness of breath (SOB) when at rest or with exertion, chronic fatigue, edema, lung crackles and distended jugular veins. CHF patients need frequent bathroom breaks because they use diuretic drugs to increase urinary output and decrease fluid buildup and swelling.

## Stroke

A **stroke** (cerebrovascular accident or CVA) is a sudden stoppage of blood flow to the brain. Strokes occur because a blood clot causes blockage (known as a cerebral embolism), or a blood vessel in the brain bursts (known as a cerebral hemorrhage). Vessel tissues in the brain die and cause a cerebral infarction. Signs and symptoms of stroke include severe headache, speech loss, dizziness, weakness or paralysis on one side of the body (hemiplegia), and loss of consciousness. If a patient experiences a stroke in the dental office, terminate the procedure. Remove all instruments from the mouth. Raise the patient's head slightly. Call EMS. Give oxygen by mask. Check vital signs until EMS arrives. Cardiopulmonary resuscitation may also be necessary.

## Impact of Kidney Disease on Oral Health

**Chronic kidney disease** can have multiple effects on dental health.

- If the kidneys are not functioning properly, patients may complain of a bad taste or bad smell in their mouth. This occurs due to the kidneys not removing urea from the blood. Urea breakdowns to form ammonia, which causes halitosis, or bad breath.
- The renal system is also responsible for the absorption of calcium. If calcium is not being absorbed appropriately, the teeth and bony structures can become weakened, which contributes to tooth loss and breakdown of the bony structure of the jaw bones.
- Patients who are undergoing dialysis treatments may receive a blood thinner in their shunt at the time of their treatments. For this reason, dental procedures should be scheduled on a day in which they are not undergoing dialysis. This decreases the risk of excessive bleeding during dental procedures.
- Chronic kidney disease impairs the function of the immune system, which can increase the risk of infection following even routine dental work. These patients are usually given an antibiotic to take before any dental work is performed.

## TREATING PATIENTS WITH LIVER DISEASE

The most common **liver disorders** that affect dental health are hepatitis, alcoholic and non-alcoholic liver cirrhosis, and hepatocellular carcinoma. The liver produces many of the proteins essential in appropriate blood clotting. Excess bleeding can be a common problem during dental procedures on patients with liver disease.

- *Hepatitis C* commonly causes lichen planus, an inflammatory condition that causes painful lesions in the mouth, and xerostomia, a condition that results in dry mouth and increases the risk of tooth decay. Sialadenitis, or inflammation of the salivary glands, can also result in dryness within the mouth causing tooth decay and gum disease.
- *Jaundice* is present when the liver is not breaking down old red blood cells which results in elevated bilirubin levels. This buildup of bilirubin within the skin and other soft tissues can result in yellow discoloration of the gums and oral mucosa.
- Dental personnel should also exercise increased caution with patients who have a *viral form of hepatitis* due to the risk of contracting the disease through contact with blood. The disease cannot be spread through exposure to infected saliva.

## NEUROLOGICAL DISEASE AND DENTAL HEALTH

**Neurological diseases** can affect dental health through disorders of nerves in the head and oral cavity, as well as through the inability to perform daily oral hygiene activities due to lack of nerve and muscle control.

- Conditions such as *strokes* or *neurologic trauma* can impair a person's ability to perform appropriate oral hygiene to prevent tooth and gum disease due to paralysis.
- *Parkinson's disease* affects a person's ability to maintain adequate control of mouth movements, which can lead to difficulty in providing adequate oral hygiene. The spasticity associated with Parkinson's disease can also lead to teeth grinding and disorders of the temporomandibular joint.
- Patients with *epilepsy* or other *seizure disorders* can suffer broken and cracked teeth during seizure activity.
- Dental abnormalities are also seen in patients with *multiple sclerosis*. The loss of muscle control and the spasticity associated with this disease can impair a person's ability to maintain adequate oral hygiene through brushing and flossing.
- Patients with forms of *dementia* may not be able to perform personal hygiene, which can lead to tooth decay and gum disease.

## MEDICAL CONDITIONS AND ASSOCIATED DENTAL CONCERNS

| Medical condition | Dental concerns |
| --- | --- |
| Emphysema, COPD | Patient may need to sit upright to relieve shortness of breath and may use pursed-lip breathing, making it difficult to keep the mouth open. Rubber dams should be avoided. The patient may cough and expectorate frequently and may have an infection, therefore dental personnel may need to wear masks. Treatments may need to be done intermittently at short intervals. If the patient has severe shortness of breath, an upper respiratory infection, and/or oxygen saturation level of <91%, the appointment should be rescheduled. |
| Hypertension | The patient's blood pressure may increase with the stress of dental care, so it's necessary to provide a calm environment and to reassure the patient. Any medications the patient is on should be noted as they may affect the dentist's choice of treatment. The blood pressure should be monitored with any complaint of headache or dizziness. |
| Rheumatic fever | Preventive antibiotics are no longer recommended for patients with a history of rheumatic fever unless they have had infective endocarditis or other heart complications. Otherwise, routine care is indicated. |
| Hypotension | Hypotensive patients may experience a further drop in blood pressure with anxiety, causing the patient to faint or experience dizziness; but hypotension may also indicate an allergic reaction or other medical complication, such as a heart attack, so for patients who report hypotension, the blood pressure should be monitored carefully. |
| Pregnancy | Pregnancy and the weeks of gestation must be noted as some medications and treatments must be avoided because of danger to the fetus. Gums may be prone to bleeding due to pregnancy gingivitis. X-rays should be avoided if possible but any taken should be done with thyroid collar and lead apron. In later stages of pregnancy, the patient may become hypotensive if placed in supine position. Elective dental care is usually avoided during the first trimester. |
| Respiratory infection | Patients may expose others to infection through coughing, so patients should be rescheduled if possible. If not, then the dental personnel should all wear facemasks and carry out careful hand hygiene. |

## PATIENTS AT RISK FOR BACTERIAL ENDOCARDITIS

**Bacterial endocarditis** is inflammation of the lining of the heart caused by a bacterial infection. Patients with a history of congenital heart disease or rheumatic fever are very susceptible to bacterial endocarditis. People who have had heart valve replacements, joint replacements, or organ transplants are also predisposed to development of bacterial endocarditis. An individual with a heart murmur is at risk for endocarditis. Insertion of dental implants also puts patients at risk. Any patient with one of these risk factors should be given a broad-spectrum antibiotic prior to dental treatments or procedures to avoid infection. The recommended standard prophylactic course of therapy for adults is pre-procedure oral amoxicillin V (3 gm 1 hour before), erythromycin stearate (1 gm 2 hours before) or Clindamycin (300 mg 1 hour before) followed by half doses 6 hours later. Doses for children depend on body weight: 50 mg/kg amoxicillin, 20 mg/kg for erythromycin, or 10 mg/kg for Clindamycin given 1 hour before procedures, followed by half doses 6 hours later.

## HYPERVENTILATION

**Hyperventilation** is deep and rapid breathing, usually as a result of anxiety. The patient who hyperventilates for a prolonged period becomes faint, loses feeling in the extremities, and cannot take complete breaths. Alkalosis (high blood pH) further exacerbates the anxiety and rapid breathing. Terminate the procedure. Sit the patient erect. Allay the patient's anxieties. Instruct the patient to hold his or her breath a few seconds before exhalation, which reverses the alkalosis by getting more carbon dioxide and less oxygen into the blood. Alternatively, have the patient breathe into a paper sack or their hands.

The converse is shallow breathing or **hypoventilation**, which can result in $CO_2$ accumulation in the blood and needs supplementary oxygen by mask.

## FOREIGN BODY AIRWAY OBSTRUCTION

A dental patient is reclined, anesthetized, and slippery objects are in the mouth, so there are many opportunities for **foreign body airway obstruction (FBAO)** to occur. The universal distress signal for FBAO is clutching of the throat with both hands. If the patient does this, suspend treatment immediately. A choking patient cannot speak. Breathing is difficult or absent. The mouth may be blue (cyanotic). Ask the patient to sit up and cough. If he/she cannot force out the foreign body independently, call for help. Perform the Heimlich maneuver to open the blocked airway. If the patient is conscious, stand behind him/her. Wrap arms around the abdomen. Make one hand into a fist; grasp the other hand firmly over it. Deliver a series of swift subdiaphragmatic thrusts, until the airway is clear or the patient falls unconscious. The patient needs follow-up medical treatment in case the airway was damaged.

## ABDOMINAL THRUSTS FOR UNCONSCIOUS PATIENT WITH AIRWAY OBSTRUCTION

If a patient with foreign body airway obstruction (FBAO) becomes **unconscious** during the standing Heimlich maneuver, call Emergency Medical Services (EMS) immediately. Brain death occurs in 4 to 6 minutes. Place the patient on his or her back. Don gloves. Lift the tongue and jaw and check if the foreign body is visible. If so, attempt to remove the foreign body manually. A blind finger sweep is no longer recommended, therefore if no foreign body is visible, open the airway by tilting the head, lifting the chin, pinching the nose. Insert a resuscitation mask into the mouth. Blow two slow breaths into the airway. Repositioning of the head may be required. If the airway remains obstructed, then landmark the xiphoid process. Straddle the patient's thighs. Position the heels of both hands just below the xiphoid notch at the base of the sternum. One hand is on top of the other. Apply 5 abdominal thrusts, pressing toward the diaphragm. Continue thrusting until the airway is unblocked or EMS arrives to take over.

## SYNCOPE

**Syncope** is fainting, loss of consciousness from decreased blood flow to the brain and blood pooling in the extremities. Syncope is caused by stress, pain, shock from massive infection or drug reactions, or standing for too long. The patient faints because lying down restores blood flow to the brain. The patient feels dizzy or nauseated, initially. Lower his or her head to increase blood flow to the brain. If unconscious occurs but the patient is breathing normally, place him/her in the Trendelenburg position (lying back with slightly elevated feet), so blood streams back to the brain. If the patient does not breathe well, open the airway by inclining the head and raising the chin. Remove restrictive clothing (scarves or ties) or jewelry at the neck. Dispense oxygen, using an oxygen tank, mask, and tubing. If breathing does not resume in 15 seconds, remove the oxygen mask. Apply spirits of ammonia under the patient's nose with a gauze sponge for a second or two. The unpleasant fumes should stimulate the person to take in air and oxygen and revive within a minute. Call an ambulance and start CPR, if necessary.

## SIGNIFICANT BLOOD LOSS

The patient who experiences significant **blood loss** needs intravenous fluid and electrolyte replacement, and perhaps a blood transfusion. If the dentist books a procedure where hemorrhage is likely, then the Blood Transfusion laboratory crossmatches the patient beforehand. Two units of blood are reserved in the laboratory's refrigerator, in anticipation of hemorrhage. For example, males with hemophilia or Christmas disease and females with von Willebrand disease may need immediate transfusions, additional clotting factors, and IV fluids. Book a registered nurse to assist with the procedure. The blood group (A, B, AB, or O) and Rh type (negative or positive antigen) of both donor and recipient must match before transfusion. A fatality can occur from mismatched blood causing hemolysis. Postpone the dental procedure if an exact match cannot be found. O– individuals are universal donors, in great demand. AB individuals are universal recipients (the rarest and most difficult group to match).

## ULCERS

Many **oral ulcers** or sores are not contagious and can be soothed with topical anesthetics. Cold sores are contagious, and are caused by herpes simplex virus type 1 or 2 (HSV1 and HSV2). Herpetic lesions are vesicles filled with fluid containing virus. Lip clusters of these sores are termed herpes labialis. Herpes viruses attach to nerve cells and remain in the body for life. Herpes virus is usually dormant, but is reactivated by exposure to stressors or acidic food. The dental team should avoid contact with cold sores. Reschedule the patient if lesions are present, if possible. If procedures must be performed during an active infection, topical treatments can provide some relief. Wear gloves and other PPE. If the patient's vesicles break, the dental worker can get crusty ulcerations on his or her hands called herpetic willow.

## PATHOGENIC ORAL VIRUSES AND FUNGI

The **herpes** family causes most oral viral infections:

- *Herpes simplex type I* is primarily a mouth ulcer but can be transmitted by oral sex. Herpes simplex type I is contracted by physical contact in childhood. Eruptions occur throughout life. Burning vesicles are followed by crusted cold sores on the lips or in the mouth. Wear PPE when treating herpetic patients because ulcers can be developed on the hands and eyes if infected.
- *Herpes simplex type II,* the genital variety, can appear in the mouth.
- *Herpes zoster* is shingles and usually affects the elderly. It is a reactivation of childhood Varicella (chickenpox). Herpes zoster lesions are usually one-sided along the course of a nerve, very painful, and long lasting.

**Candidiasis (thrush)** is a thick, white monilia yeast infection coating the mucous membranes of breastfeeding children and immunosuppressed patients. Gently scrape the plaque. Apply topical antifungals. AIDS patients may have chronic Herpes simplex, Herpes zoster, and thrush infections, causing weight loss.

## PRECAUTIONS AGAINST HIV CARRIERS

The **human immunodeficiency virus (HIV)** is transmitted via sexual intercourse, from mother to fetus, or through transfusion with infected blood products. The retrovirus replicates in the immune cells called T-lymphocytes, so they cannot alert the body to infection. Some HIV carriers are asymptomatic, while others have ambiguous conditions like weight loss, night sweats, or diarrhea. HIV infection precedes AIDS, acquired immunodeficiency syndrome, characterized by dementia and opportunistic infections like thrush, pneumonia, and Kaposi's sarcoma. AIDS is incurable but there are now several classes of drugs that slow its effects, including reverse transcriptase and protease inhibitors. Life expectancy has risen from 18 months to 10 years for many AIDS patients. The most commonly used drugs are zidovudine (AZT) and acyclovir. Universal precautions apply to treating patients with HIV. Dental personnel must wear PPE (gloves, gown and mask) and avoid contact with body fluids of patients with HIV or AIDS.

## PRECAUTIONS AGAINST VIRAL HEPATITIS CARRIERS

**Hepatitis** is inflammation of the liver, characterized by jaundice, abdominal pain, fever, and weakness. Hepatitis A and E are caused by contact with contaminated food or water, and usually just produce temporary flu-like symptoms. People with Hepatitis A are treated with gamma globulin injections or the Havrix vaccine. Hepatitis types B, C and D are bloodborne. Hepatitis B is quite virulent and some forms are fatal in 14 days. All dental personnel should be vaccinated against it with Heptavax-B, Recombivax HB, or Engerix B in a sequence of three injections. Hepatitis C is less virulent but more chronic; vaccine development is impeded by its mutational ability. Both Hepatitis B and C may present asymptomatically, as jaundice, loss of appetite, abdominal discomfort, fever, muscle pain, or weakness. Hepatitis D can only replicate in conjunction with Hepatitis B. Dental personnel must wear PPE and avoid contact with body fluids of patients with hepatitis.

## LUMPY JAW AND SYPHILIS

**Lumpy jaw** is an abscess caused by a bacterial infection, called actinomycosis. The usual culprit is the anaerobic bacterium Actinomyces israelii. Actinomyces species are commensal mouth and throat flora that neither hurt nor help their host. However, after surgery or trauma, Actinomyces can become a pathogen that causes swollen, reddish-purple lumps, pus-draining skin sores with yellow "sulfur" granules, fever, and weight loss. Lumpy jaw produces little or no pain. The dental assistant swabs the sore for culture and sensitivity testing. The doctor may lance the lump. The patient needs antibiotics for several months up to one year to clear actinomycosis. Left untreated, it infects the lungs and causes sores on the chest wall.

**Syphilis** is a venereal disease transmitted by sexual or mother-to-fetus contact with Treponema pallidum spirochetes. Syphilis has three stages:

- Lip chancres (firm, raised lesions that develop ulcers and crusting).
- Infectious patches or papules.
- Localized gummas or tumors.

Children of syphilitic mothers have tooth enamel hypoplasia, or Hutchinson's incisor's (ragged incisal edges), or mulberry molars.

## POORLY MANAGED ORAL HEALTH AND SEPSIS OR SHOCK

Poor oral health can lead to decayed and broken teeth. This exposes the pulp of the tooth, which can become infected. The pulp contains the blood vessels, connective tissue, and nerves of the tooth. If the infection spreads from the pulp into the blood vessels of the tooth, it can be carried throughout the body and lead to a condition called sepsis. **Sepsis** results in tissue damage, organ failure, and can even cause death if not treated promptly.

By performing adequate oral hygiene, the risk of dental infection is greatly reduced, which can also decrease the risk of developing sepsis as a result of a dental infection. Having regular dental checkups can also help to prevent dental infections that could lead to sepsis. With the use of x-rays and oral photography, the dentist can detect any conditions within the teeth that could potentially lead to infection. Early gum disease can also be identified using these techniques, which will also decrease the risk of oral infections.

## LOOSE PERMANENT OR TEMPORARY CROWNS

In addition to anatomical and clinical definitions of crown, the term also refers to prostheses that cover the coronal surface of a tooth with broad decay or other problems. There are full-cast crowns that enclose the complete coronal surface and partial crowns that cover up to three tooth surfaces. They are usually made of porcelain, gold, stainless steel, or a combination of porcelain and metal. **Loss of a permanent or temporary crown** is a dental emergency. A temporary fix is to use petroleum jelly or orthodontic wax to keep the crown in position. The individual must be careful during meals not to dislodge the crown. As soon as possible, the crown should be recemented in place with the appropriate type of cement.

## PROSTHETIC REPLACEMENT

The **loss of a dental prosthetic** is considered a dental emergency because of the effect it can have on speech and eating. Repair or replacement of a broken or lost prosthetic is considered as important as the loss of a tooth.

The **process of replacement** a dental prosthesis depends upon the type of prosthesis being used. These can be removable appliances, such as dentures, or fixed prosthetics, such as dental implants. In either case, a mold of the patient's oral structures is taken to ensure the prosthesis will fit properly within the mouth. Once the prosthetic is created based upon the patient's existing oral structures, a final fitting is performed with alterations made as necessary for a removal prosthesis. This ensures that a denture, for example, will fit properly without being too loose or too tight. Dental implants are replaced through oral surgery involving the placement of a post within the jaw bone that will hold the artificial tooth, or teeth, in place.

## DENTAL PULP VITALITY TEST

The **dental pulp vitality test** is used to assess the pulp, dental nerve, and blood flow of the pulp and roots of a tooth. It can be used to evaluate whether there is a dental abscess present, whether the pulp is necrotic, or if the tooth is normal.

An electric or thermal (hot or cold) stimulus is applied to the tooth to be evaluated. The stimulus is slowly increased until the patient feels sensation within the tooth. The neighboring teeth are also usually tested, along with the contralateral tooth. If the patient does not notice a change in sensation as the stimulus is increased, there is usually necrosis (death) of the pulp or a dental abscess present. If the patient experiences an immediate sensation when the stimulus is applied, inflammation of the pulp is usually present which usually eventually leads to necrosis. If the stimulus elicits a change in sensation that is equal to the neighboring teeth, the tooth in question is usually healthy without any disease present.

# Substance Use

## WARNING SIGNS FOR USE OF MARIJUANA OR COCAINE

Two widespread abused drugs are **marijuana** and **cocaine**.

Patients who have taken **marijuana** recently may have an extremely high heart rate. The active ingredient is tetrahydrocannabinol (THC), but marijuana is often dusted with contaminants, so it is equally a stimulant and depressant. Habitual use damages lungs and reproductive organs. Chronic marijuana users have problems with memory, speech, coordination, and lack of motivation. Currently there is no evidence of physical dependence on marijuana, but users become emotionally dependent on it. Marijuana reduces nausea in cancer patients and reduces eye pressure in glaucoma patients. Marijuana has been legalized in states across the country for various levels of use: some only for medical use, and recreational use recently legalized in others.

**Cocaine** is addictive both physically and psychologically. It is often combined with other addictive drugs, potentiating its effects and the possibility of drug interactions. It is a stimulant and numbs the mouth. Cocaine abuse leads to cardiovascular issues, extreme anxiety, violent conduct, mental illnesses, and death.

## WARNING SIGNS FOR TOBACCO, CAFFEINE OR ALCOHOL USE

**Tobacco, caffeine, and alcohol** are readily available and legal for adults. However, all these drugs are addictive. Smokers and tobacco chewers are stimulated by nicotine, which predisposes users to lung, bladder and oral cancer, heart disease, stained teeth, gum damage, and halitosis. Moderate consumption of caffeinated drinks (coffee, tea, chocolate, maté, guarana) is safe, but excessive consumption overstimulates the heart and nervous system, creates stomach ulcers, and stains teeth. Alcoholic beverages contain ethyl alcohol, a depressant, which slows reflexes and leads to poor judgment, coordination, and speech. Chronic alcohol abuse lead to dependency, convulsions, delusional behavior, and cirrhosis of the liver.

## ORAL LESIONS CAUSED BY TOBACCO USE

Use of tobacco is the main **chemical cause of oral lesions**. Nicotine stomatitis is common in pipe smokers and, to a lesser extent, cigarette smokers. Mouth areas repeatedly exposed to the heat and chemicals in tobacco initially redden from irritation. Later, they develop white and red, thick bumps containing keratin protein (hyperkeratinized). The patient's salivary gland openings may also become inflamed. Another type of tobacco-related lesion can occur with use of snuff or chewing tobacco. The lesion occurs generally in the lower front mouth, between lips and teeth, and is similar to nicotine stomatitis. Irritations from smoking marijuana can look very similar to tobacco use, although marijuana lesions usually occur inside both lips.

## CHEMICAL AGENTS OTHER THAN TOBACCO THAT CAN CAUSE ORAL LESIONS

Hairy tongue (lingua villosa) is lengthened, darkened tongue papillae. A thick coating covers the tongue's middle dorsum, especially near the throat. It may be black brown, green, white, or pink. Papillae wave if they are shot with a blast of compressed air. Causes include: **Broad spectrum antibiotics; tobacco; intravenous drugs; coffee; tea; breath mints; candies; hydrogen peroxide rinses; low fiber diet; poor oral hygiene; and HIV.** Signs include halitosis (bad breath) because long papillae trap food, and gagging or tickling when the patient swallows. Instruct the patient to brush his or her tongue and eliminate the agents to cure hairy tongue.

The seizure medication **phenytoin (Dilantin),** orthodontic braces, or plaque can cause gingival hyperplasia. Connective tissue from the gum extends over the teeth, affecting eating and appearance. If the irritant (e.g., an essential drug) cannot be removed, surgical removal is an option.

Patients who put **acetylsalicylic acid (ASA)** over aching roots develop Aspirin burn, in which coarse, white lesions form.

## WARNING SIGNS FOR USE OF HALLUCINOGENS

**Hallucinogenic drugs** are drugs of abuse. They cause a user to imagine events, people, or things that are not really present. Subsequently, the user has modified brain activity, causing unpredictable or violent behavior. LSD (lysergic acid diethylamide) and its close relative psilocybin are both hallucinogens. LSD is derived from the fungus ergot and psilocybin comes from mushrooms. Phencyclidine (PCP) is another hallucinogen that has both stimulatory and depressive effects, like violent conduct, convulsions, nausea, suppressed respiration, and prolonged memory loss. Mescaline, derived from the peyote cactus, does not promote such extreme behavior, but it can cause permanent psychosis. If the dental assistant suspects that the patient is abusing a hallucinogen, treatment should be suspended and the dentist notified.

## WARNING SIGNS FOR AMPHETAMINE OR BARBITURATE USE

**Amphetamines** and **barbiturates** have opposite effects, but both are addictive.

- **Amphetamines** are stimulants, increasing heart and respiratory rates and blood pressure. Aggressive behavior and poor judgment are warning signs of amphetamine use. Amphetamines do have an accepted medical use in treatment of narcolepsy or for attention deficit hyperactivity disorder (ADHD).
- **Barbiturates** slow down brain activity and have a calming or tranquilizing effect. Phenobarbital is administered for insomnia, epilepsy, and anxiety (including in the dental office). The main issues with barbiturates are dependency and tolerance with long-term use, withdrawal symptoms if taken away after prolonged use, and potentially critical overdosing. Overdosing causes disorientation, coma and death.

# Drugs and Drug-Induced Emergencies

## USE OF NARCOTIC DRUGS WITHIN CONTEXT OF DENTISTRY

**Narcotic drugs** are depressants that have the potential for physical and psychological addiction. Two narcotics, morphine and codeine, are often administered as analgesics (pain killers). Morphine is for severe pain and may be administered intravenously, intramuscularly, or orally. Occasional use causes constipation, nausea, and disorientation. Habitual use leads to addiction. Codeine is for mild to moderate pain, usually in formulations with Aspirin or acetaminophen. Its main side effects are tiredness and constipation. Heroin has no accepted medical use. It is taken intravenously, subcutaneously, or via inhalation. Heroin addicts develop tolerance to high doses. Warning signs of heroin use are depressed respiratory and heart rates, constipation, and loss of appetite. A heroin overdose is an emergency situation, characterized by vomiting, diarrhea, shock, and loss of consciousness. Call EMS to transfer the overdosed heroin addict immediately to a hospital, where he/she can be given a narcotic antagonist.

## DRUG SIDE EFFECTS, DRUG INTERACTIONS, AND DRUG ADDICTION

Drugs are chemicals that alter bodily processes, treat diseases, or alleviate pain. They are naturally-occurring or artificially created. Laws require certain drugs to be dispensed only by prescription, while others can be obtained over-the-counter (OTC). The only professionals licensed to write prescriptions for controlled substances are doctors, dentists, and physician assistants. The benefits of drugs must be balanced against their side-effects and drug interactions. **Side-effects** are inadvertent consequences of use of a particular drug. For example, the immunosuppressant drug cyclosporine, which thwarts organ graft rejection, makes the patient susceptible to infection. **Drug interactions** are unintentional consequences of simultaneous use of two or more drugs. The combination of drugs acts synergistically to magnify, diminish or change the effects of each. **Drug addiction** means physical dependency on a drug and withdrawal symptoms if it is discontinued.

## DRUG ADMINISTRATION ROUTES

These are the **routes of drug administration** in the dental office:

- *Oral* as pills or liquids for prophylactic antibiotics.
- *Topical administration* for anesthesia (ointment or cream applied to the skin or oral mucosa).
- *Gas inhalation*, particularly nitrous oxide.
- *Injections*: Intravenous (into the vein for rapid response); intramuscular (into muscle); subcutaneous (underneath the skin) or intradermal (between skin layers).
- *Sublingual* (under the tongue, as with nitroglycerine and fentanyl).
- *Transdermal skin patch*, releasing medication at a steady rate, as with nitroglycerine cream or nicotine patch.
- *Rectal administration* of suppositories or enemas may be applicable for patients at home before or after the procedure, e.g., Gravol for nausea or fentanyl for severe pain in cancer patients.

## CURRENT DRUG LAWS

The **Food and Drug Administration (FDA)** controls drugs. Drug laws relevant to dental practice are the 1906 Pure Food and Drug Act, the 1938 The Pure Food, Drug, and Cosmetic Act, and especially the Comprehensive Drug Abuse Prevention and Control Act of 1970, which divides drugs into **five schedules**, based on their potential for abuse:

- *Schedule I drugs* - Great potential for abuse and no established medical benefit, such as heroin.
- *Schedule II drugs* - Great possibility of abuse and dependence but with some known medical benefit, e.g., narcotics, opiates, some barbiturates, and amphetamines.
- *Schedule III drugs* - Less potential for abuse and established medical utility; includes other barbiturates, stimulants, strong depressants, and combinations, including many drugs used in dental practice.
- *Schedule IV drugs* - Some potential for abuse, with established medical utility, and little possibility of addiction; includes sedatives, anti-anxiety drugs, and certain depressants.
- *Schedule V drugs* - Slight potential for abuse; dispensed over-the-counter.

## POSSIBLE COMPLICATIONS WITH TOPICAL OR LOCAL ANESTHETIC

**Topical anesthetics** can cause allergic and toxic reactions. Swelling, erythema, ulcerations, and difficulty swallowing or breathing up to a day or more after application indicate an allergic reaction, which should be treated with antihistamines. Toxic reactions are central nervous system (CNS) complications due to an overdose of topical anesthetic. The patient initially becomes talkative and anxious. His or her blood pressure and pulse rates increase, but later the patient becomes hypotensive and the pulse is weak and thready. Excessive administration of local anesthetic drugs can produce similar toxic reactions and paresthesia (numbness). Document reports of paresthesia because nerve damage can be permanent.

## ANTIBIOTICS

**Antibiotics** treat bacterial infections. Broad-spectrum antibiotics kill many microorganisms, including helpful normal flora. Penicillin, and its derivatives amoxicillin and ampicillin, are broad-spectrum antibiotics. An antibiotic can only kill organisms that are sensitive to it; many organisms are now resistant due to overuse of antibiotics. Antibiotics can cause allergic skin or respiratory reactions, which are treated with antihistamines. Common antibiotic side-effects are nausea, diarrhea, and yeast infections due to disruption of normal flora. Prophylactic ampicillin taken 2 hours before teeth scaling prevent heart complications (for bacterial endocarditis) in patients who had rheumatic fever. The penicillin derivative oxacillin is for Staphylococcus aureus infections. Penicillin G is only for Gram-positive bacteria. People with penicillin allergies are generally given erythromycin, instead. Tetracyclines are antibiotics that discolor emerging teeth and precipitate kidney failure.

## ANTICHOLINERGIC DRUGS, ANALGESICS, AND TRANQUILIZERS

**Anticholinergic drugs** block nerve impulses. They reduce lung secretions while the patient is under general anesthesia, treat bradycardia, and dilate the pupils of the eyes. Dentists give anticholinergics to inhibit the patient's salivation while an impression is made. The drugs of choice are atropine sulfate or propantheline bromide. An **analgesic** is a drug that relieves pain but does not cause unconsciousness. Non-narcotic analgesics include ibuprofen and acetaminophen; they are for mild to moderate pain. Narcotic analgesics produce stupor and sleep and are for moderate to severe pain. Dental narcotics include morphine sulphate and meperidine hydrochloride. Aspirin is avoided because it inhibits healing due to its blood-thinning and clot-suppressing qualities. It also irritates the stomach. **Tranquilizers**, particularly diazepam (Valium), are often given prior to procedures to relax anxious patients.

# Patient Management and Administrative Duties

## Patient Management and Communication

### EFFECTS OF PSYCHOLOGY, COMMUNICATION, AND LISTENING SKILLS ON PATIENT MANAGEMENT

**Psychology** is the study of the mind and people's characteristic mental makeup. Each person brings an acquired belief system (paradigm) to his or her interactions with others. Patients have preconceived ideas about dental practices. Many are apprehensive about pain. The dental assistant must understand paradigms and employ good communication and listening skills to facilitate successful patient interaction and management.

**Communication** is the exchange of information. Good communication consists of skillful interpretation of the message by the sender (in this case the dental professional), interpretation of the message by the receiver (the patient), and establishment of a connection, as indicated by feedback. **Active listening** on the part of both sender and receiver enhances good communication.

### VERBAL AND NONVERBAL COMMUNICATION SKILLS

Any type of communication between people that does not involve words is **nonverbal communication**. Up to 93% of successful communication depends on nonverbal cues. Remember that a dental patient is unable to speak during a procedure and is likely apprehensive. Watch the patient's facial expressions, gestures, posture, and position. Tight posture and/or crossed arms and legs suggest resistance. Conversely, relaxed posture and uncrossed appendage suggest openness. The dental assistant's posture affects the patient. Sit close to the patient, rather than towering directly over him/her in an intimidating manner. Maintain the proper social distance (territoriality) between oneself and the patient during discussions (~3 feet). A patient feels more comfortable when he/she is well-informed beforehand and the professional works from the side.

### MULTI-CULTURAL COMMUNICATION

Different **cultures** have different value systems, and the dental professional must be aware of these to ensure a successful practice. Realize that social distance, eye contact, and use of first names versus surnames differs among cultures. For example: Arabs find a social distance of 2 feet best; Asians find direct eye contact rude; Israelis talk on a first-name basis; and in Hispanic cultures, the oldest male family member speaks for the patient. Familiarize oneself with the immigrant population in the area and take diversity training. The American Dental Association offers Spanish explanations of common procedures at http://www.ada.org/public/espanol/index.asp. Know where to find interpreters who understand dental terminology. Book the interpreter at least a day before the procedure. Speak slowly while facing the patient; do not address the translator first. Try to get more than perfunctory feedback from the patient during the communication.

# Oral Health Information

## KEY TOPICS IN PEDIATRIC AND ADULT PATIENT EDUCATION

Key topics in patient **dental education** include:

- *Pediatrics*: Children should be shown how to brush their teeth, how often, and for how long (usually at least 2 minutes) and shown how to use dental floss. They should also be advised to brush or drink water after eating sweets and to chew sugar-free gum. Older children should be instructed about the importance of a mouthguard when playing sports. Children who will have braces need to understand how the braces align the teeth, how the braces are applied, and how to care for them.
- *Adult*: In addition to the above, adults need to be educated about the effects of aging on dental health and ways to prevent gum disease. They should be advised regarding various options for dental care, including whitening and other cosmetic procedures as well as the importance of routine teeth cleaning. More specific information should be provided for any dental procedures, such as root canals.

## ORAL HYGIENE FOR PATIENTS WITH SPECIAL NEEDS

All **patients with special needs** require empathy and individual attention from the dental professional. The nausea that usually accompanies pregnancy presents problems related to oral hygiene. Acid regurgitated from the stomach during bouts of nausea promotes decay, the act of tooth brushing often causes gagging, and the women commonly have bleeding gums. Advise pregnant patients that these circumstances may occur, and suggest they perform dental hygiene when they are not nauseated. Cancer patients commonly experience xerostomia (mouth dryness), widespread caries (including the roots), gum bleeding, and deficient muscle function. Approaches to oral hygiene issues include use of topical fluoride and/or extra-soft or foam toothbrushes. Patients with heart disease experience similar problems. Patients with arthritis may need to use special large toothbrushes or floss holders.

## DIETARY SOURCES OF ENERGY

All food consumed by an individual is his diet. Nutrients are dietary chemicals, essential for growth, maintenance and healing. There are six classes of nutrients. Three are **energy sources**: Carbohydrates, fats, and proteins. The other three classes are vitamins, minerals and water. Carbohydrates (sugars, starches, and fibers) provide energy, so at least half of the diet should be carbs. Fats and lipids are water-insoluble and contain fatty acids. Fat insulates, transports Vitamins A, D, E and K, and provides energy when sugars are inaccessible. Proteins are linked amino acids. Proteins derive from plant and animal sources, and are vital for cell growth and repair. Of 20 possible amino acids, 10 are manufactured by the body and 10 are essential and must be provided in the diet. Animal proteins (eggs, milk, meat) contain all essential amino acids and are complete. Plant sources do not contain all essential amino acids and are incomplete. Different incomplete foods eaten in the same meal are complementary (e.g., beans and rice) and provide complete nutrition.

## RELATIONSHIP BETWEEN CALORIE CONSUMPTION AND EXPENDITURE

**Consumed calories** provide energy. Carbohydrates supply 4 Calories (C or Cal) per gram consumed, fats 9 Cal/gram, and proteins 4 Cal/gram. A person's rate of metabolism is the relationship between bodily changes and energy expenditure. Everyone has a resting or basal metabolic rate (BMR). BMR is higher in children, thin people, and expectant women. The primary energy source is carbohydrates, while fats are also utilized when sugars are inaccessible. Conversely, if calories are not used, they are converted to fat and stored. Both carbohydrates and fatty acids comprising fats are made of the elements carbon, oxygen and hydrogen, in different configurations.

## MINERALS

**Minerals** are elements that cannot be broken down chemically. Seven major elements and a few trace elements are required to sustain life. Minerals with negatively or positively charged ions are electrolytes.

- Two major minerals, *calcium* and *phosphorus*, are important for development of bones and teeth and are necessary to prevent osteoporosis. Calcium is involved in muscle contraction, conduction of nerve impulses and blood clotting. Phosphorus is involved in energy transfer and pH balance. Milk and cheese are good sources of calcium and phosphorous.
- *Sodium* and *potassium* are complementary major minerals that maintain fluid balance in the blood. Sodium, found in table salt and processed foods, causes high blood pressure in excess. Table salt also contains the mineral chlorine, which helps pH balance.
- *Sulfur* is important because it is a necessary component of protein and plays a role in metabolism of energy.
- *Magnesium*, found mostly in green vegetables and whole grains, also affects energy metabolism.

## DIETARY TRACE MINERALS

Some minerals are found in the body in small or trace amounts. Fluorine, which is necessary for strong teeth and to avert osteoporosis, is considered a trace element. Numerous **trace minerals** facilitate metabolic processes, including iodine, copper, chromium, selenium, manganese, and molybdenum. Iodine is unique in that is concentrated in the thyroid gland. The trace mineral iron is a carrier of oxygen in blood; a deficit of iron can cause anemia. Cobalt is also necessary for red blood cell maintenance. Zinc is required by the immune system and promotes tissue growth.

## CARIOGENIC FOODS

Carbohydrates contain the chemical elements carbon, hydrogen and oxygen, and are comprised of sugars, starches and fibers. Carbohydrates from natural sources include fruits, grains, and legumes. Most naturally-occurring carbohydrates are not broken down to simple sugars until they arrive at the stomach. **Cariogenic foods** are converted to simple sugars right in the mouth, where bacteria change them into acids. The acid demineralizes the enamel, predisposing the teeth to caries (decay). Manufactured sweets, such as candies and soft drinks, and naturally-occurring raisins and sticky fruits do are cariogenic. The dental assistant should evaluate the patient's diet for use of cariogenic foods. Explain the possible consequences to the patient. The acid from cariogenic foods can be somewhat neutralized if they are eaten with foods that stimulate saliva production. Conversely, eating cariogenic foods late at night, when saliva production is low, enhances potential decay. New teeth in infants are susceptible to nursing bottle syndrome, rampant decay due to liquid sweets, such as fruit juice.

## WATER-SOLUBLE VITAMINS

Vitamin C and B complex are **water-soluble**. Vitamin C (ascorbic acid) is found in all citrus fruits and vegetables, like tomatoes and broccoli. Vitamin C is a necessary component of collagen, needed in connective tissue. It prevents scurvy, aids wound healing, and helps tooth development. Vitamin B complex includes:

- *Thiamine (B₁)*, essential as a coenzyme in the oxidation of glucose and to avert the degenerative nerve disease beriberi.
- *Riboflavin (B₂)*, which aids growth, energy release from food and protein production.
- *Niacin (B₃)* or nicotinic acid, needed for ATP synthesis and maintains the gastrointestinal and nervous systems.
- *Pyridoxine (B₆)*, which plays a role antibody, nonessential amino acids, and niacin production.
- *Biotin (B₇)* and *pantothenic acid (B₅)*, which help with energy metabolism.
- *Folate (B₉)*, which is involved in RBC production.
- *Cobalamin (B₁₂)*, which synthesizes red blood cells (RBCs) and maintains myelin sheaths.

## FAT-SOLUBLE VITAMINS

Nutrients that carry out essential functions but are not energy sources are vitamins. Four vitamins are **fat-soluble** and retained in the liver and other fatty tissues, Vitamins A, D, E and K. Vitamin A is available as carotene in dark leafy vegetables and orange or yellow fruits, and from dairy products and liver. It is essential for maintenance of mucous membranes, bones, skin (epithelial tissue), and vision. Vitamin D or cholecalciferol is necessary for good bone and tooth growth. It is available in animal sources, such as eggs, liver, and fortified milk. It can also be produced in the body after ultraviolet ray or sun exposure. Vitamin E or alpha tocopherol is obtained via plant sources, such as avocadoes, wheat germ, almonds, and fortified margarine. It is an antioxidant that prevents other nutrients from breaking down. Vitamin K is found in green leafy vegetables and animal products, like milk, liver, and egg yolks. Its primary function is to stimulate the formation of prothrombin, which is involved in blood clotting and coagulation.

## DEFICIENCIES OR EXCESSES OF VITAMIN INTAKE

All vitamins in proper amounts have beneficial effects. Vitamin A **deficiency** causes night blindness and inadequate bone growth. Vitamin D deficiency causes rickets, osteomalacia, and inadequately developed teeth. Vitamin $B_2$ or $B_6$ deficiencies cause mouth fissures and inflammation of the tongue. Vitamin C deficiency causes scurvy with tooth loss and muscle cramps. Vitamin E deficiency causes RBC destruction. Vitamin $B_{12}$ deficiency causes pernicious anemia.

Conversely, fat soluble vitamins, C, $B_3$ and $B_6$ are toxic if consumed to **excess**. Too much Vitamin A causes stunted growth and termination of menstruation. Vitamin C or D toxicity results in kidney stones. Vitamin E toxicity causes hypertension. Vitamin K toxicity causes hemolytic anemia or jaundice. Excess niacin causes rash and liver damage. Excess $B_6$ damages nerves. High amounts of other water-soluble vitamins are not toxic because they are excreted in the urine every four hours.

## NORMAL OCCLUSION

**Occlusion** is the relationship of the upper and lower teeth to each other when they are touching, such as when eating or at rest. Maintaining normal occlusion of the dental structures is important to prevent further problems. Occlusion can become abnormal from missing teeth, crowded teeth, crooked teeth, poorly fitting crowns or other prosthetics, or abnormal jaw growth.

If these problems are not corrected early in life, they can go on to cause serious problems with oral health. These problems include weakened ligaments, muscles, and tendons of the jaw that can impact the ability to speak and eat. The patient can develop pain through the teeth. The teeth can also become excessively worn down or can fall out if the malocclusion is severe enough. The gums can also be affected with recession of the tissue at the gum line due to poor occlusion of the dental structures. Chronic pain can develop in the temporomandibular joint due to problems with occlusion.

## MALOCCLUSION

In 1890, Edward Angle described a **classification system for grading the degrees of malocclusion**. These degrees are based on the relationship between the mesiobuccal cusp of the maxillary first molar and the buccal groove of the mandibular first molar.

- *Class I:* The relationship of the molars is normal, but there is crowding and misaligned teeth. This results in a minor overbite and is often corrected for cosmetic purposes.
- *Class II:* The buccal groove of the mandibular first molar is distally positioned when in occlusion with the mesiobuccal cusp of the maxillary first molar. This causes a severe overbite and can contribute to tooth decay, gum disease, and worn tooth enamel.
- *Class III:* The buccal groove of the mandibular first molar is medially positioned when in occlusion with the mesiobuccal cusp of the maxillary first molar. This can cause a severe under bite and can contribute to tooth decay, gum disease, and worn tooth enamel. This can also lead to TMJ syndrome.

## FLUORIDE

**Fluoride** is a mineral derivative of the element fluorine. Fluoride is primarily absorbed via the gastrointestinal tract, and is found in low amounts in normal bone and dental enamel. Fluoride incorporated into tooth enamel forms fluorapatite crystals. Optimal fluoride exposure should be between 0.7 and 1.2 ppm, giving the teeth a gleaming, white, unblemished appearance. Average fluoride levels are lower in teeth with caries. If high amounts of fluoride are ingested during tooth development, the child's teeth acquire a mottled appearance, known as fluorosis. Excessive fluoride causes either chronic or acute fluoride poisoning. Chronic fluoride poisoning occurs from habitual ingestion, usually through a fluoridated water supply. Teeth mottle with a fluoride content up to 1.8 ppm. Enamel hypocalcifies at1.8 to 2.0 ppm of fluoride, so teeth are chalky, with discolored bands, flecks, cracks, and pits.

### BENEFICIAL EFFECTS

**Fluoride** can reduce dental caries because it binds to the bacteria in plaque, thus retarding acid production and decay. Fluoride can remineralize soft areas and reverse very early tooth decay. Dentists and hygienists administer gel or foam fluoride in trays to reinforce children's teeth once or twice yearly. Topical fluoride only accesses the outer enamel layer.

| Systemic Sources of Fluoride | Topical Sources of Fluoride | |
|---|---|---|
| Fluoridation of the water supply with 0.7 to 1.2 parts sodium fluoride per million parts water. | 2% Sodium fluoride | Professionally applied |
| Ingestion of meat, cereals, and citrus fruits. | 8% Stannous fluoride | |
| Prescription tablets, drops, lozenges, or vitamin preparations given to children up until their second molars erupt. | 1.23% Acidulated phosphate fluoride | |
| | Dentifrices (toothpastes) | Self-applied |
| | Polishing pastes | |
| | Mouth rinses | |

## SALIVA

**Saliva** performs 4 main functions:

- *Cleanses the mouth.* Saliva keeps the mouth moist and aids in washing bacteria and food off the teeth and oral mucosa. This can help to prevent gum disease and tooth decay. It also helps to prevent halitosis, or bad breath.
- *Dissolves food chemicals.* Saliva helps to dissolve the chemicals in food to improve taste, such as breaking down salt and other seasonings. This can help to stimulate the appetite and ensure adequate intake of calories for overall health.
- *Moistens food.* The saliva helps to compact the chewed food into very small pieces so that it can be formed into a bolus. Once the bolus is formed, the food can be more easily swallowed to travel through the rest of the digestive system.
- *Breaks down food.* Saliva contains enzymes that begin the digestive process of certain foods. Carbohydrates are the first food group to be broken down and this process begins within the mouth due to enzymes that breakdown starches.

## PRIMARY AND PERMANENT TEETH

**Primary teeth,** or "baby" teeth, help children to chew, speak, and smile. They support the lips and surrounding oral mucosa. They hold spaces in the jaws through which the permanent teeth will erupt. They also make it easier for the tongue to form words by serving as a brace against which the tongue can push when forming certain letter sounds. The function that primary teeth play in speech development is extremely important at a young age.

**Permanent teeth,** or "adult" teeth, help primarily with chewing food, but they also serve a role in articulating speech. Depending upon which type of permanent teeth is chewing, they are responsible for biting, tearing, crushing, and grinding food to aid in digestion. Correct placement of the permanent teeth is imperative for proper speech development and word formation. The correct placement of permanent teeth is also necessary for forming normal occlusion of the teeth to prevent tooth decay and gum disease.

## GOOD PREVENTIVE DENTISTRY

**Good preventive dentistry** is multifaceted. It involves daily brushing and flossing for removal of plaque and bacteria. Teach the patient correct techniques for brushing and flossing at the initial visit. It is advisable to use a disclosing agent at regular intervals to see how successful the removal has been. Children who are still developing dentition should undergo a fluoride program, including treatments at the office and in the home. A healthy patient should see the dentist every six months. Routine visits should include an examination, cleaning, and dental procedures, if indicated. In addition, good nutrition and adequate exercise have a positive impact on general health, including teeth and bones.

## DENTAL PLAQUE

**Dental plaque** is a tacky, bacteria-containing mass found on teeth that have not been brushed thoroughly. It looks like a soft, white, sticky accumulation. It is concentrated near the gingiva. The bacteria feed off consumed sugar and convert it to acid. The acid, in turn, damages the tooth enamel by causing demineralization. The content of the minerals calcium and phosphate is depressed. Demineralization on enamel surfaces looks chalky and white. Demineralization is often a problem found in patients who have had orthodontic appliances removed where the brackets were previously situated. Eventually, plaque that is not removed leads to tooth decay.

## PLAQUE DISCLOSING AIDS

**Plaque disclosing aids** are used to identify areas on the surface of the teeth that contain plaque. It is usually a solution or a tablet that is given to the patient. After the disclosing aid is used, areas of the teeth will be stained a different color to identify the plaque. Plaque has the ability to absorb the stain readily, which causes it to become discolored when the disclosing aid is used.

Plaque disclosing aids are useful to assist the dental professional in locating the specific areas that will require more care during a dental cleaning. They plaque in these areas can then be removed through a thorough dental cleaning. Patients may be given the plaque disclosing solution or tablets to use at home in order to evaluate the thoroughness of brushing and identify the areas of the mouth that may require more attention. This can also be used to motivate patients and allow them to see the progress they are making when performing their own dental care at home.

## ORAL HYGIENE AIDS

**Oral hygiene aids** include disclosing agents, dentifrice, toothbrushes, flosses, mouth rinses, chewing gum, and a variety of interdental aids. Dentifrice is another term for toothpaste, used by the patient with a toothbrush or floss. Dentifrice products earn the ADA Seal of Acceptance if they are deemed both safe and effective. Toothpastes contain abrasive materials, and often fluoride for decay prevention, or other ingredients (for example whiteners or calculus inhibitors). Mouth rinses are designed to be swirled in the mouth to dislodge debris or temporarily get rid of halitosis, as adjuncts to brushing and flossing. Some have ingredients (alcohol) that eradicate microorganisms. Special oral hygiene gums chewed after eating carbohydrates encourage saliva production and loosen debris. Interdental aids clean between the teeth and stimulate the gums. They include the interproximal brush, dental stimulators, floss holders and threaders, and irrigators.

## INTERDENTAL AIDS

Interdental aids are described below:

- **Interproximal brushes** consist of a handle (often bent) attached to a small, nylon-bristled brush. They reach into interproximal areas, open bifurcations and trifurcations, and under orthodontic brackets. Dental stimulators activate soft tissues in interproximal areas and get rid of plaque.
- Some toothbrushes have rubber tipped stimulator ends. **Wooden dental stimulators** made of balsam wedges have plastic handles with toothpick tips attached; moisten both before use.
- **Floss holders** are "Y" shaped to hold floss for easy access to interproximal areas. Shift the floss up and down on the sides of the tooth and into the sulcus.
- **Floss threaders** are rigid plastic, shaped into a large loop at one end, through which floss is threaded. Insert the straight end into one side of the space. Pull it out the other for removal, leaving the floss for elimination of plaque and debris.
- A **water irrigation device** uses pulses of water to remove debris. Irrigators are for cleaning orthodontic brackets and prostheses and are ineffective against plaque.

## DENTAL FLOSSING

**Dental flossing** removes plaque and fragments from proximal tooth surfaces. Traditional dental floss comes as a thread that is either waxed or unwaxed. Waxed floss glides more easily and is less likely to tear or snag. Flosses can be flat tape, finely textured, colored, or flavored. Flossing requires 18 inches of floss. Secure the ends around the middle and ring fingers of each hand. Grasp a short section (about an inch) between the thumb and index finger of each hand. Draw the floss into each proximal space, using a gentle back-and-forth motion. In the maxilla, use both thumbs or a thumb and finger. For the mandible, use the two index fingers. The floss should be wrapped around the proximal surface and into the sulcus. Move the floss up and down along the surface for plaque removal. Transfer it to the proximal surface of the adjoining tooth, and repeat the action. Use a new section of floss for each space. Include the distal surface of the last molar.

## TOOTHBRUSHES

All **toothbrushes** fall into two main categories: Manual or mechanical.

- *Manual toothbrushes* have a head containing the bristles, an indented shank adjacent to the head, and a long handle. There may also be a rubber dental stimulator on the end. The head has a toe end at the exterior and a heel end at the interior. Bristle configurations differ on various brushes; they are usually spaced or multi-tufted. Manual toothbrushes with soft, nylon bristles are best because they are durable and will not wear away the teeth or gums.
- *Mechanical toothbrushes* are attached to a recharging unit or are battery operated. Their heads t can move in various directions: Reciprocating (back and forth), vibratory (quick back and forth), orbital (circular), arched (in a semi-circle), elliptical (oval rotation), or a combination of movements. Mechanical toothbrushes may also include sonic action.

## BASS AND MODIFIED BASS MANUAL TOOTH BRUSHING TECHNIQUES

The main objective of **tooth brushing** is the thorough cleaning of every surface of all teeth. Manual brushing should take 2 to 3 minutes. Manual brushing techniques include the Bass, modified Bass, Charter, modified Stillman, rolling stroke, and modified scrub-brushing techniques. Dentists most often recommend the Bass or modified Bass techniques because they are effective at removing plaque near the gums.

- **Bass technique:** Hold the toothbrush bristles slanted at 45° to the teeth, toward the gingival sulcus. Sequentially brush small areas, each for a count of 10, with small back and forth movements. Apply the toe bristles to the lingual surfaces of the front teeth.
- **Modified Bass technique**: Essentially the same, except after each area has been cleaned, bring the bristles are up over the crown toward the biting surface.

## CHARTERS AND MODIFIED SCRUB-BRUSHING TECHNIQUES

Charters and modified scrub brushing techniques are effective for plaque removal and gum stimulation.

- With the **Charters brushing technique**, the toothbrush head is pointed toward the end of the root. The brushes touch the gingiva, centered between adjacent teeth, and are aimed toward the teeth. Small areas are sequentially brushed for a count of 10 each, with small back and forth movements. Front teeth are brushed with the sides of the toe bristles and the brush parallel to the teeth.
- The **modified scrub brushing technique** uses back-and-forth movements centered initially between the gum and tooth. The brush is held perpendicular to the tooth surface. This is repeated until all teeth have been cleaned.

## Modified Stillman and Rolling Stroke Brushing Techniques

Modified Stillman and rolling stroke-brushing techniques are effective for plaque removal and gingival stimulation. In both, the initial position of the bristles is toward the apex of the tooth.

- The **modified Stillman method** also positions the handle level with the biting surface. The bristles are brushed downward simultaneously, with a back-and-forth action, to cover the complete surface of the tooth for a count of 10. The patient performs a minimum of 5 sequences before continuing to the next tooth and repeating the sequence.
- With the **rolling stroke brushing technique**, the toothbrush is held parallel to the tooth, with the bristles toward the apex. The bristles are rolled from the gums down toward the teeth, including the biting surface. Each tooth is brushed in this manner 5 times before moving to the next one. A similar motion is applied on the lingual surfaces of the front teeth, using either the toe or heel portion.

## Evaluating Patient's Response to Home-Care Therapy

The GCA can **evaluate the patient's response to home-care therapy** through subjective and objective information.

- *Subjectively*, the patient can describe their symptoms. If they were having dental pain related to a specific problem before, it is hoped that their pain has decreased. It is important to ask the patient whether they have been having any difficulty with performing any interventions at home to help their problem. Identifying any obstacles the patient is having to complete home-care therapies can help to increase compliance and improve outcomes.
- *Objectively*, the oral exam can provide information on how a specific problem appears. If the home-care therapies are being performed appropriately, there should be improvement in the appearance of the problem. Referring back to oral photographs that were taken before treatment started can provide a "before and after" reference to visualize improvement. These can also be shared with the patient so they can see the improvement they have attained through the treatments they have performed at home.

## Pre- and Post-Treatment Instructions

**Pre-treatment instructions**: For surgery, advise the patient to remove contact lenses and wear loose clothing that allows for monitoring of blood pressure and to avoid taking aspirin for a week prior to surgery, other NSAIDS for 2 to 3 days, and alcohol for 12 hours before surgery. If the patient is to be sedated, the patient must have an adult to drive to and from the appointment.

**Post-treatment instructions**: For cosmetic restoration, advise the patient to expect some difficulty speaking and increased saliva for a few days. With crowns, advise the patient to return to the office if the crown loosens or comes off. Following extractions, advise the patient to keep pressure (gauze plug) on the site for 30 to 40 minutes or longer if bleeding persists and to notify dentist for prolonged or severe bleeding. Once a clot forms, the patient should avoid drinking from straws, smoking, and rinsing forcefully or brushing teeth about extraction site for 72 hours. After fillings, advise the patient to avoid eating or drinking hot liquids until numbness subsides.

## Traits of Infants and Children That Can Impact Oral Health

The **oral health of infants** is the responsibility of the parent or guardian. The adult removes the infant's plaque with an infant toothbrush or cloth while the child reclines. Instruct parents to bring the child to the dentist at **age 3 years old**. Preschoolers respond to visual instruction but they also have a short attention span. Role-play to teach the child oral hygiene habits. Tell the parent to oversee or perform tooth brushing at bedtime. **Children ages 5 to 8** have a longer attention span and are eager for knowledge. They can be taught good oral hygiene techniques with visual aids, like short videos or pictures. **Children ages 9 to 12,** have an even longer attention span, greater curiosity, and the ability to brush and floss effectively on their own. They also have unique issues, such as peer group acceptance and dealing with mixed dentition, which the dental assistant should keep in mind when providing instruction.

## TRAITS OF TEENAGERS, ADULTS, AND OLDER ADULTS THAT CAN IMPACT ORAL HEALTH

Peer pressure and concern about personal appearance motivate all teenagers. **Thirteen to fifteen-year-olds** have poor coordination (due to growth spurts) and bad eating habits. Thus, they often have trouble with flossing. The decay rate in this age group increases dramatically. The dental assistant should give individualized instructions and encouragement to motivate young teenagers. **Sixteen to nineteen-year-olds** question authority and have busy schedules. The assistant needs to act more as a friend. Explain the processes involved in plaque and caries formation. Approach **young and middle-aged adults** on an individualized basis. **Elder older than 60** have age-related concerns, such as tooth retention, disease-specific difficulties, maintaining oral hygiene with poor sight, or use of drugs that interfere with oral health. The professional needs to give advice based on each specific case.

## CARING FOR HEARING IMPAIRED OR VISUALLY IMPAIRED PATIENTS

There are many physical disabilities that must be accommodated in the dental office. **Accommodations** are discussed below:

- *Hearing impaired*: Assess the level of hearing impairment and the patient's preferred method of communication (hearing aid, writing notes, sign language, lip reading, etc.). For lip readers, be sure that the mouth is visible when speaking, and sit in a position that the patient can easily read lips. Lightly tap the patient to notify them that you are speaking. Use written explanations if there is any confusion. For sign language, utilize medical interpreter who is able to communicate all relevant information to the patient. Look at the patient when speaking, not the interpreter. Patients with hearing aids may choose to turn it off during treatment so be sure to allow them to make that decision.
- *Visually impaired:* Assess level of visual impairment. Slowly acquaint the patient to the dental office and dental treatment room. Utilize a Tell-Feel-Do technique to demonstrate and prepare patients for ongoing procedures. Avoid sudden movements or loud noises that may startle the patient.

## CARING FOR WHEELCHAIR BOUND OR NON-ENGLISH-SPEAKING PATIENTS

- *Wheelchair bound*: The Americans with Disabilities Act (ADA) Standards for Accessible Design (2010) requires that dental offices offer a barrier-free environment for individuals that are wheelchair bound. Guidelines require reserved parking spots for patients in wheelchairs, sidewalks that are 3 feet wide, at least one entrance that is wide enough to accommodate wheelchair entrance and is on ground level or accessible by ramp, dental treatment rooms that can accommodate wheelchair entrance and storage in addition to the personnel and equipment required, and a dental chair that can be lowered to 19 inches above the ground for easy transfer to and from the chair.

- *Non-English speakers*: The most recommended accommodation when treating patients that are non-English speakers is the use of a professional interpreter. Dental offices with high levels of non-English speaking patients may have an onsite interpreter or access to interpreters by phone. Other alternatives include visual models and diagrams, videos, brochures, or in non-emergent situations, informal interpreters such as family may be utilized (though this is not encouraged in the case of consent and when making decisions that should prioritize the patient's input and best interest).

## ADVANTAGES AND DISADVANTAGES OF RESTORATIVE MATERIALS/PROCEDURES

**Restorative materials and procedures** in dentistry are performed to correct structural problems with the teeth. This can include a composite filling, crowns, bridges, dentures, and implants.

The main advantage of restorative procedures is to maintain the structure of the tooth, or teeth, to prevent impairments of eating or speech. This can also help to maintain gum health and prevent gum disease. Repair or replacement of a tooth may also help to decrease pain, which can improve the quality of life.

A disadvantage of restorative materials or procedures is the risk of malfunction or damage to the device. Crowns can come off and require the creation of a new crown. Dentures can break or become ill fitting, which may require repair or refitting of them. Implants are also subject to falling out and would need to be replaced. This requires a dental procedure with associated pain and expense. Even simple fillings can become loose and fall out, which would require they be replaced.

## PROPER CARE FOR REMOVABLE APPLIANCES AND PROSTHESES

**Removable dental appliances or prostheses** come in the form of dentures, which can be partial or complete. Cleaning and caring for the appliance are the same regardless if it is partial or complete.

- After eating, rinse the dentures with water to remove any pieces of food.
- Be careful to avoid dropping the dentures because they can break. Placing a towel on the counter or in the sink when cleaning will help to protect them in case they are dropped.
- After removing dentures, a soft toothbrush should be used to gently clean the gums, oral mucosa, and tongue.
- Dentures should be brushed daily using a denture cleaner. I denture adhesive is used, be sure to completely remove the adhesive when cleaning.
- In order to help dentures maintain their shape, they should be soaked in water overnight. A mild denture cleaning solution may be used, depending upon the manufacturer's recommendations.
- Rinse the dentures well before inserting them, especially if a denture cleaning soak is used overnight.

## PROPER CARE FOR NON-REMOVABLE APPLIANCES AND PROSTHESES

Care of the two most common types of **non-removable dental appliances**, a dental bridge and implants, is similar to caring for natural teeth:

- A *dental bridge* is a dental appliance that replaces missing teeth. It is anchored to existing teeth to fill in a gap where there are missing teeth. Every day, dental floss or a specialized small toothbrush should be used to clean under the artificial teeth. This will help to remove any food or debris that is stuck underneath the bridge. Regular brushing should be performed twice daily to clean all of the teeth.

- *Dental implants* can be cared for the same as natural teeth. In order to prevent plaque build-up, a soft toothbrush should be used at least twice daily to brush the teeth. This is especially important after meals. The implants should also be flossed, the same as natural teeth.
- Regular dental checkups are imperative to have non-removable appliances and prostheses examined for any cracks or chips. The fitting of these devices should also be assessed to ensure there is not crowding from the surrounding teeth.

## EFFECT OF SYSTEMIC DISEASE ON HEALING

Any **systemic disease** that increases overall inflammation within the body and decreases tissue perfusion can have an adverse effect on oral health. For example, diabetic patients are much more likely to experience gum and periodontal disease due to circulatory impairment. Decreased tissue perfusion due to vascular changes associated with diabetes can increase the risk of developing oral disease. Heart disease also affects vascular flow, which can interfere with adequate perfusion through the gums. The increase in inflammatory markers due to chronic heart disease also increases the risk of inflammation within the oral cavity, which can increase the risk for periodontal disease and impaired healing.

Patients with **chronic disease** and associated inflammation will also have impaired healing. Decreased tissue perfusion and decreased blood flow interferes with the body's ability to fight infection by limiting the number of immune cells present in the area. Often, an oral antibiotic will be prescribed to the patient to take before undergoing any dental procedures to decrease the risk of oral infection.

## PROPER PROTOCOL FOR ORAL AND WRITTEN PRE- AND POST-TREATMENT INSTRUCTIONS

As part of the patient's right to be informed of their care, they also have the right and responsibility to prepare for and recover from their treatment appropriately in order to maximize the effectiveness of the treatment. It is the responsibility of the dental team to provide **pre- and post-treatment instructions** to the patient, both in person (orally), and through written instructions to ensure that the patient understands their responsibilities and has a reference to those instructions at home. The in-person/oral instructions allow the patient the opportunity to ask questions and for the dental team to assess understanding. In the case of patients that may have barriers in this process, accommodations should be provided, such as an interpreter and instructions in the patient's primary language, brochures with images to support the instructions, or access to a digital video with subtitles. As patients may not be best equipped to receive post-treatment instructions immediately following their treatment, both pre- and post-treatment instructions should be provided to the patient at the same time, at the appointment prior to the treatment.

# Reception, Communication and Accounting

## TELEPHONE AND BUSINESS OFFICE COMMUNICATION TECHNOLOGIES

Voicemail changed the way dental offices operate, because the system automatically routes the caller to the mailbox for a specific professional, without screening by a receptionist. The dentist and dental assistants are legally responsible for ensuring patients can access dental personnel in an emergency. Do not let an emergency caller flounder in "voicemail jail." List the numbers for the locum tenens and nearest emergency dental clinic in the outgoing message on the answering machine. Turn the machine on only when personnel are not present. Check for messages immediately upon return. An answering service operator can contact the dentist via a pager that flashes the patient's callback number. If the call is unanswered in a pre-agreed time, the service reroutes the call to the locum tenens. Healthcare professionals may carry cellular phones for direct contact, and some are capable of receiving faxes, images, and text messages. Answering services and cell phones are more expensive than voice mail, but help ensure legal compliance with duty of care.

## TELEPHONE ETIQUETTE

All personnel should be aware of **good telephone etiquette**:

- Remember, patients and visitors in the waiting room can overhear conversations, so be discreet.
- Answer all incoming calls within 2 to 3 rings.
- Identify the practice to the caller, e.g., "XYZ Dental Clinic. [Your name] speaking. How may I help you?"
- Be organized, attentive and courteous. Speak clearly and directly into the mouthpiece, pronounce words properly, and speak at a normal speed.
- Practice good listening skills.
- Obtain and use the caller's name.
- Screen the call; find out where to direct it best.
- Take a message, including date, time, caller's name, phone number, recipient's name, the communication, and callback parameters.
- Do not keep a caller holding longer than one minute.
- Reserve outgoing calls primarily for next day appointment confirmations.
- When communicating with patients whose primary language is not English, be patient, speak slowly at a normal volume, and repeat if required. Get an interpreter when necessary.

## DENTAL RECEPTIONIST AND DENTAL OFFICE BOOKKEEPER

The **dental receptionist** is responsible for initially greeting patients, helping them to fill out needed paperwork, answering the telephone, taking memos, arranging appointments, overseeing the charts and records, and other assigned tasks. The receptionist may or may not assume the role of dental office bookkeeper. The employee hired to be the dental office bookkeeper deals with all office finances, including Accounts Receivable (money owed to the practice) and Accounts Payable (for which the office owes money). The bookkeeper may also handle dental insurance, payment arrangement details, and the inventory and supply system. Many dental offices have an office manager who coordinates and provides backup for these duties.

## DENTAL ASSISTANT'S DAILY ROUTINE FOR OPENING THE OFFICE

Every morning upon **opening the office**, the dental assistant first changes from street wear into protective clothing, like a lab coat or uniform, so that external contaminants do not enter treatment rooms. The assistant then turns on the following: Lights; dental units; vacuum system; air compressor; x-ray processors; sterilizers; communication system; and computers. The assistant checks the patient schedule and performs routine housekeeping chores, like: Unlocking files; organizing the reception and business areas; replenishing water and solutions for radiographic processing; preparing disinfectant solutions; setting out trays and lab work for the first patients; and restocking any necessary supplies. The assistant finishes any overnight sterilization procedures before the dentist needs the instruments.

## DENTAL ASSISTANT'S DAILY ROUTINE FOR CLOSING THE OFFICE

Ideally, two dental assistants participate in **closing the office** every day. They need to clean the chairs and units in the treatment rooms, flush various systems, and shut off switches. They process, mount, and file x-rays, and turn off radiographic processing equipment and the safe light. One assistant sterilizes used instruments while the other sets up trays for the next day. One assistant verifies that all laboratory work was sent out, and completed lab work has been returned. They deal with assigned chores, like insurance, bookkeeping, confirming appointments, and pulling charts for the next day's appointments. They turn off all business equipment, turn on the answering machine, and bolt windows and doors. Assistants change out of their uniforms into street wear before leaving, so they do not bring contaminants home.

## PATIENT SCHEDULING

**Patient scheduling** is performed by the receptionist. Appointment books are being phased out in favor of computer software. However, all personnel should know how to schedule and cancel an appointment with the correct color-code manually and on computer, in case the system fails or requires maintenance. 10 or 15-minute blocks are allocated for expected procedures. Include some time with the dental assistant alone and in tandem with the dentist. Allow double booking when one professional is free to attend to another patient's needs. Block out dates when the dentist is unavailable throughout the year on an appointment matrix. Set aside buffer times in the morning and afternoon for dental emergencies. Schedule children around their nap times or school hours. Make considerations for patients with special needs, such as booking an interpreter or attendant.

## APPOINTMENT BOOK ENTRIES

Determine an appropriate time in conjunction with the patient. Use a pencil for **appointment book entries** to allow for changes. Enter the patient's name, phone number, age (for children), type and length of appointment. Give the patient an appointment card immediately. Familiarize the receptionist with the length of various procedures, to avoid downtime, overtime, scheduling conflicts, and double-booked treatment rooms. Schedule contagious patients at the end of the day. Sales representatives require appointments. Students must work when qualified staff is available to supervise them. If relying solely on computer bookings, print off the next day's schedule in case of computer failure.

## SYSTEMS FOR PATIENT RECALL

Patients are scheduled for continued care or **recall appointments** by one of four methods:

- Set the computer to automatically generate a recall date and inform the patient at the end of the visit. At month end, the computer generates a list of patients for recall the next month, and the receptionist contacts them.
- Schedule a tentative recall in the appointment book six months in advance while the patient is in the office, and tell him/her to confirm the appointment when the date nears.

- Ask the patient to self-address a postcard. Place it in a chronological card file by month. Mail the card to the patient two weeks before ideal recall.
- Color-code an index card with all pertinent patient information. Phone all patients with the same color code one month beforehand.

## DENTAL INSURANCE

A person who has contracted **dental insurance** is the subscriber. Anyone covered by the policy is a beneficiary. Insurance can be primary or secondary, depending on whether it is obtained via a subscriber or spouse. Group plans are offered by an employer to its employees, or by an organization to its members. Individual plans are available to members of the public. Dependents are spouses, children younger than 18 years old, or full-time college students. A carrier is the insurance company administering the plan. Carriers set annual maximums for reimbursement and deductible amounts that must be paid before benefits accrue. Predetermination of benefits is a process by which the dentist sends a proposed treatment plan to the carrier to calculate how much it will cover.

## SUBMITTING DENTAL INSURANCE CLAIMS

Each completed dental procedure is assigned a **five-digit CDT code** that begins with a D for dental. CDT codes are described in the ADA's Current Dental Terminology. The patient must endorse on the claim form their assignment of benefits, which states that the benefits should be paid from the insurance carrier directly to the dentist or other provider. In lieu of an endorsement, there is a tacit agreement that the patient will pay for services independently. A signature on file can also be used for assignment of benefits. The patient signs another area for release of information to the carrier. The form has fields for patient identification. Insurance claims can be submitted by mail or electronically. Carriers have established schedules of benefits, detailing amounts they will reimburse for various activities.

## ALTERNATIVES TO DENTAL INSURANCE

Alternatives to dental insurance include:

- **Health maintenance organizations (HMOs)** administer capitation programs, where the dentist gets a fixed fee based on the number of patients he/she serves.
- **Medicare** is an example of a contract fee schedule plan, in which dentists in the plan agree to accept defined, reduced fees for specific services.
- **Managed care plans** focus on preventive care and limit the procedures that can be performed or medications that can be prescribed.
- **Direct reimbursement plans** do not use an insurance carrier as an intermediary; here the patient pays for services and then is refunded money by his or her employer, who is the plan administrator.

## USUAL, REASONABLE, AND CUSTOMARY PATIENT FEES

Dental offices set up a **fee schedule** for specific services rendered. Fees charged are defined as usual, reasonable, or customary.

- The *usual fee* is that normally charged by the dentist.
- A *reasonable fee* is one falling in the midrange charged, based on the procedure and difficulty.

- The *customary fee* reflects local averages up to the 90th percentile. Insurance companies will not reimburse amounts above what they have determined to be usual, reasonable and customary. When a dentist charges less, for example, as a professional courtesy or for a limited insurance program, there is no source to recover the rest of the usual, reasonable or customary fee.

## BOOKKEEPING INVOLVED IN ACCOUNTS RECEIVABLE

The dental office bookkeeper handles **Accounts Receivable** and Accounts Payable, either by computer software or the manual pegboard system. Computerized systems have all pertinent patient information, description of services, charges, payments, and insurance information organized and easily accessible. The account status can be viewed or printed out. The pegboard system uses day sheets that list patient names and all procedures, charges and receipts for that day. No-carbon-required paper is used. There are columns for balancing all daily and individual patients' Accounts Receivable. Total amounts received daily are deposited promptly in a bank account. Patients are invoiced monthly. Partial or deferred arrangements are extended to patients with good credit ratings.

## ACCOUNTS PAYABLE

**Accounts Payable** responsibilities are assigned to the bookkeeper or office manager. Some functions that require clinical knowledge, such as inventory supply and control, are assigned to the dental assistant. The total amount of Accounts Receivable (A/R) is the practice's gross income. Accounts Payable (A/P) is money paid out for various expenses. Deduct the A/P from the gross income to determine the net income or profit. Permanent salaries, mortgage payments, and utilities are steady fixed expenses. Monthly expenses that change, such as supplies or repairs, are variable expenses. The combination of fixed and variable expenses is the practice's overhead. Once or twice monthly, the dentist authorizes payment of Accounts Payable. There may be petty cash kept at Reception to cover incidental costs, like taxi couriers.

## REFERRALS

There are several reasons why a dentist would **refer** a patient to an oral surgeon:

- Impacted teeth that require cutting into the gum tissue or the bony tissue of the jaws.
- Insertion of the post that is rooted into the jawbone for dental implants. Once it is healed, the dentist will affix the artificial tooth onto the post.
- Decreased bone mass in the jaws or the need for strengthening of the jaw.
- Decreased bone mass in the upper jaw can be corrected by an oral surgeon in order to prevent sinus complications from dental implants.
- Jaw disorders resulting from infection, trauma, or TMJ disorders.
- Repair of broken or lost teeth due to trauma, along with treating associated trauma to the gums.

When referring a patient to an oral surgeon, the patient's face sheet, insurance information, and progress notes from their dental office visit should be forwarded to their office. Any x-ray images or dental photographs should also be included. The dentist may want to include additional correspondence explaining the purpose for the referral or any concerns they may have.

# Legal Records

## PATIENT RECORDS

A **patient record** is a legal document containing pertinent information related to the individual and his or her care. Patient records should be retained for at least seven years from the last visit and kept confidential. On the left, attach the Registration Form for demographics, such as: Patient name; address; phone numbers; employer; spousal or parental information; payer; insurance, if any [photocopy the insurance card]; and chief complaint. On the right side, attach a Medical History, including: Prescription, over-the-counter, and street drugs; exposure to radiation and toxins; medical conditions (e.g., diabetes, epilepsy, pregnancy, bleeding disorders, or rheumatic fever); allergies marked with brightly-colored alert stickers; and height and weight to calculate anesthetic dose. The dentist authorizes the Dental History form. The patient or guardian signs and dates Consent to Treatment and Release of Information forms, for legal coverage and continuity of care. Keep the patient record in reverse chronological order, with the most recent treatment record on top and the oldest at the bottom.

A patient's dental record must be correct and current because it is a subpoenable court document that may be reviewed by a judge, prosecutor, defense lawyers, and privacy commissioner. The dentist may be required to appear in court to explain their documentation. Document all care and payments legibly in ink. If a mistake is made, never use correction fluid or an eraser to fix it. Strike through the original entry with one line. Write the correct information above it. Initial and date the change. Keep records at least seven years from the last service date. Most dentists keep them indefinitely because of variations in the statute of limitations, the time period for local legal action. Place a signed informed consent in the chart for any surgical procedures. The dentist must explain the procedure, risks, expected results, alternatives, and perils associated with denying treatment before asking the patient to sign the informed consent form. Implied consent is an implicit contract between dentist and patient whenever the latter allows work to be performed.

### FORMS AND HISTORIES

If the patient has any conditions that require the dentist to consult with the physician, then ask the patient to sign a **Release of Information form.** Before subsequent visits, ask the patient's doctor to complete a **Medical History update form**. Include laboratory reports for communicable diseases. The diseases of concern are hepatitis and human immunodeficiency virus (HIV/AIDS). Give the patient (or his or her guardian) a written description of the right to privacy under the Health Insurance Portability and Accountability Act (HIPAA). Keep these signed forms for at least 7 years from the last visit. Document the examination, dental charting, and oral radiography. The dentist reports suspicious lesions or other medical conditions (e.g., suspected heart disease) back to the physician.

## DENTAL RECORDS MANAGEMENT

Keep **dental records** in color-coded file-folders. File cabinets must be locked when unattended to comply with privacy laws. The most popular type of file cabinet used in dental offices is the open-shelf lateral file cabinet, in which files can be pulled out. Vertical file cabinets are often used. Files must be sorted alphabetically, starting with the last name, proceeding to the first name, and lastly the middle name. Patient information sent via computer or facsimile must be protected from hackers. Keep records indefinitely. Microfilm records older than seven years. Keep a tickler file containing index cards with tasks that should be completed by a certain time. Alternatively, set a computer reminder to perform the tasks.

## STORING IMAGES, HISTORIES, AND CORRESPONDENCE

The proper processes for storing images, histories, and correspondence in patient records are as follows:

- **Images:** If electronic records are utilized, the x-ray system is usually synced with the records to allow images to be downloaded into the patient chart. If hard copies of x-ray films are being stored, they should be kept in a climate-controlled area that will minimize damage to the films. Digital photographs should be downloaded into the patient's electronic health record if this is available.
- **Histories:** The dental and medical history should be gathered from the patient at their initial appointment and at least annually after that. Generally, at every visit, the patient should be asked if there has been any change to their medical history or medications. This information should be documented in the patient's chart.
- **Correspondence:** Correspondence from specialists that may be utilized for referrals should be kept in its own section of the chart so it can be found easily. Any correspondence to the patient regarding their care should also be included in the patient chart. Documentation pertaining to billing or account delinquency should not be kept in the medical chart.

## MANAGING SECURITY RECORDS FOR CONTROLLED SUBSTANCES

Rules and regulations for the **proper documentation and storage of controlled substances** in the office are established by the Drug Enforcement Administration (DEA). These include:

- Maintain records for the purchase and wasting of all controlled substances. These need to be kept for 2-5 years depending upon state requirements.
- Controlled substances should be stored in a locked metal cabinet or safe within a locked room or closet, and bolted or cemented to the wall/floor so it cannot be removed. Access to the locked site should be limited to only a couple of personnel.
- Federal law requires a full drug inventory every 2 years, though it is advisable to keep a log book that records intake and output of any controlled substances in the office.
- Documentation should be thorough in the patient's chart pertaining to the administration of any controlled substances. Any documentation in the chart should be able to be verified through documentation in a written drug inventory log that lists the patient's name, patient identifier, drug name, and quantity given.
- When wasting a controlled substance, DEA form 41 must be completed before the drug is destroyed. Preferably, a reverse-distributor should be used.

## SHARING MEDICAL RECORDS

Under HIPAA regulations regarding privacy and security, a patient's records cannot be shared with other dental offices or healthcare providers without the permission of the patient, who must sign a release form indicating which records are to be shared and with whom. The patient should be advised of the method of sharing (paper, electronic) and the reason for sharing.

# Legal Responsibilities and Regulations

## AMERICAN DENTAL ASSISTANTS ASSOCIATION'S CODE OF PROFESSIONAL CONDUCT

There are 17 pledges that members of the American Dental Assistants Association (ADAA) subscribe to in their **Code of Professional Conduct**. The pledges are primarily related to ethics. Many of these relate to the relationship between the dental assistant and the Association, such as the dental assistant will:

- Abide by the bylaws and regulations.
- Maintain loyalty to the Association.
- Follow Association objectives.
- Respect members and employees, serve, and act cooperatively with them.
- Refrain from spreading malicious information regarding the ADAA.
- Utilize sound business principles related to the organization.
- Serve the Association and instill public confidence in it.
- Uphold high personal standards of conduct.
- Hold separate personal opinions from those endorsed by the ADAA.
- Refrain from acceptance of compensation from other members.
- Try to influence relevant legislation in a legal and ethical way.

## ETHICS

**Ethics** are moral principles or values indicative of the times. The American Dental Association's Principles of Ethics outlines the values that dental care providers must adopt to stay in practice. The main ethical concerns relate to advertising, professional fees and other charges, and the responsibilities and entitlements of the dentist relative to the patient. Dental advertising is presently considered ethical, providing it is truthful. Up until the 1980s, advertising was considered crass. Ethical behavior related to professional fees and charges means the firm's billing must conform to what other local dentists charge, the charges must be correct, and insurance dealings and missed appointments can be charged. Current ethics dictate that the dentist cannot refuse to see a patient based on discrimination against race, religion, or HIV status. HIV-infected dentists must limit their work to procedures and techniques that will not infect others. It is unethical for the dentist to be swayed by financial gains.

## STATE DENTAL PRACTICE ACTS AND BOARDS

Every state has a **Dental Practice Act**, which outlines the legal constraints and controls, which the dental team members must follow. Each state has a board that administers the Dental Practice Act, usually the State Board of Dental Examiners or the Dental Quality Assurance Board. The state board issues a dentist, a hygienist, and usually a dental assistant, a license to practice in that state only if they meet certain minimum qualifications. These requirements include educational qualifications, moral requirements, and successful completion of a written examination. A license to practice can be used in another state if the two states have a reciprocity agreement. The board defines reasons for suspension or revocation of a license. The Dental Practice Act and the corresponding board define which expanded functions a dentist can delegate to a dental assistant. Most often, the Doctrine of Respondeat Superior is invoked, making the dentist ultimately responsible, but leaving the employee accountable, too.

## ADA

In 1990, the federal **Americans with Disabilities Act (ADA)** was passed by Congress. It mandates that people with disabilities cannot be discriminated against in terms of employment and access to public services, accommodations, and goods. ADA provided more sophisticated telecommunication services to facilitate the hearing and speech impaired. ADA requires dental offices to have ramps, entryways, and treatment rooms that provide access and accommodate the needs of the disabled. The office must have at least one accessible room where patients in wheelchairs can be positioned for dental procedures. Technically, ADA applies to facilities with more than 15 employees, but all dental offices should strive to comply with ADA.

## OSHA STANDARDS

There are currently no specific **OSHA standards** for dentistry, however, there are several OSHA standards for general industry that can apply to dental practice. These include:

- *Blood borne pathogens:* Prevention of exposure to blood and body fluids.
- *Hazard communication:* Hazard warnings on container labels and safety data sheets.
- *Personal protective equipment:* Gloves, gowns, masks, face shields.
- *Medical services and first aid:* Available to employees in case of injury.
- *Ionizing radiation*: Protection against exposure to radiation at work.
- Maintenance, safeguards, and operational features for exit routes.
- Sanitation.
- *Occupational exposure to hazardous chemicals in laboratories:* Establishes a Chemical Hygiene Plan that educates employees in protecting themselves from hazardous chemicals in the lab.
- *Formaldehyde:* Educates employees on the potential hazards when working with formaldehyde, protective measures that can be taken to decrease the risk of exposure, and steps that should be taken in case of a formaldehyde exposure.
- *Forms/documentation:* OSHA requires that businesses that employ more than 10 employees must report any serious work-related injuries to OSHA.

> **Review Video: What is OSHA (Occupational Safety and Health Administration)**
> Visit mometrix.com/academy and enter code: 913559

## CDC GUIDELINES FOR INFECTION CONTROL AND PREVENTION

The **CDC guidelines** for standard precautions should be used to comply with infection control and prevention requirements.

- *Hand hygiene:* Wash hands with soap and water if they are visibly soiled. Otherwise, an alcohol-based hand rub may be used. Hands should be cleaned after touching instruments that may be contaminated, before and after treating each patient, and before and after wearing gloves.
- *Personal protective equipment (PPE):* Wear gloves with risk for contact with blood or other body fluids, mucous membrane, skin that is not intact, or contaminated equipment. Wear protective clothing with risk of clothing being soiled by blood or other body fluids. Wear a mask, face shield, and eye protection with risk for splashing of blood or other body fluids. PPE should be removed before leaving the work area.
- *Sharps safety:* Never recap needles using both hands. Use a one-handed scoop technique or syringes with retractable needles. All sharp objects should be disposed of in a sharps container that is labeled as a biohazard risk.
- *Sterilization/disinfection of instruments:* Always follow manufacturer guidelines to properly disinfect and sterilize reusable dental instruments.

# HIPAA

**HIPAA** is the federal Health Insurance Portability and Accountability Act of 1996. Congress ratified HIPAA to safeguard electronic healthcare communications, including claims, funds transfers, eligibility and claims status inquiries and replies. HIPAA directed the Department of Health and Human Services (HHS) to implement national standards for clerical and financial electronic transmissions related to healthcare. Dentists and all other healthcare providers and health plans must comply with HIPAA's privacy standards by protecting health information and the patient's rights. To find out the latest guidelines for dental offices, parameters related to use and disclosure, enforcement and preemption, visit http://www.hipaa.org/.

## PHI

**Protected health information (PHI)** is any patient identifier, such as name, Social Security number, birth date, or address. Cover all records in the reception area, so they cannot be seen by patients and visitors. Lock up unattended records. Play quiet background music to blur phone conversations, and be discrete. Place computer screens and fax machines out of patient viewing areas. Disguise names with bar codes, so the individual cannot be identified, before open transmission. Each dental office appoints a **privacy officer (PO)** who is responsible for informing patients about their privacy rights. HIPAA grants patients the right to access and copy their own dental information. Each dental office must have a written PHI policy, including requirements for use and disclosure of patient information and procedures for handling grievances. Information released to third parties must be preauthorized by the patient and kept to a minimum. Violations of PHI under HIPAA are punishable by up to $250,000 in fines and 10 years imprisonment.

## STAFF MANUAL

The staff manual must include **HIPAA's minimum requirements**:

- Table of contents.
- Identify the privacy officer (PO) in charge of informing patients about their privacy rights.
- Job descriptions of all personnel, to establish who has access to patient's information.
- Privacy policy statement.
- HIPAA training plan with training schedule.
- Copies of HIPAA forms regarding compliance, documentation, and the scheme for reporting violations.
- Confidentiality agreements between the dentist and patient.
- Agreements between the office and business associates, such as dental laboratories, computer services, records shredder, temporary employment agencies, and trash removal company.
- Contingencies for change.

## COMPUTERIZATION

Most dental business office systems are at least partially **computerized**. Networked personal computers (PCs) are connected to a secure server that complies with HIPAA. The computer programs most used are for word processing, x-ray imaging, spreadsheets, accounting, and database management. Microsoft Works, ABLEdent, Dentrix, and DentiMax are examples of common dental office software. Database management is particularly important in a dental office because these programs store vital patient contact and insurance information, track and analyze data. The practice needs an Internet Service Provider (ISP), antivirus software, a firewall, and an e-mail account regularly monitored by the receptionist.

## SAFETY ISSUES RELATED TO COMPUTER USE IN THE OFFICE

**Dental office computers** must comply with HIPAA regulations. Safeguard against computer viruses and hackers with regular antivirus and firewall updates. There must be an audit trail or another way to ensure only authorized personnel access patient records. Back up data daily to disc or external hard drive. Off-site storage is safest, in case of fire or flood. Computer operators must practice good ergonomics to avoid repetitive strain injuries, like carpal tunnel. Position the monitor with the top just below eye level and at a slightly backward incline. Position the keyboard at a height that allows for relaxed shoulders and flat wrists. Sit in a chair with lumbar supports, armrests low enough that they are not used during keyboarding, and a shallow seat to permit leaning backwards. Sit with thighs at or just above the knees, feet firmly planted on the floor, and head directly over your shoulders. Protect from eyestrain with an anti-glare screen and by looking away from the computer for 10 minutes every hour.

## DENTAL JURISPRUDENCE, CONTRACTS, AND TORTS

**Jurisprudence** is the legal system set up and enforced at various governmental levels. Laws that pertain to dentistry are referred to as dental jurisprudence. There are both civil and criminal laws. Civil laws are more often invoked in the dental setting, as they pertain to either contracts or torts.

A **contract** is an enforceable covenant between two or more competent individuals. An agreement between a dentist and his or her patient is a contract. It can be an expressed contract, with written or verbal terms, or it can be an implied contract, where actions create the contract.

**Tort law** governs the other branch of civil law. Torts relate to standards of care and wrongful actions that cause injury to a patient. Criminal laws speak to crimes that endanger society in general. There are occasions when criminal law may apply to dentistry, usually resulting in fines, incarceration, and discipline by the state dentistry board.

## LEGAL ASPECTS OF STANDARD OF CARE

**Standard of care** is covered by tort laws. Dental specialists are expected to provide due care, the accepted reasonable and judicious care. Malpractice is professional misconduct, resulting in failure to provide due care. Most malpractice lawsuits are related to professional negligence, the failure to perform what is considered standard care. Tort laws pertain to unethical or immoral behavior by the professional, resulting in harm to the patient. Examples are defamation of character, invasion of privacy, fraud, and assault and battery. Defamation of character harms an individual's character, name, or reputation through untrue and malicious statements, either written (libel) or spoken (slander). Invasion of privacy is unsolicited or unauthorized exposure of patient information. Fraud is intentional dishonesty for unfair or illegal gain. Assault is declaring one's intent to touch a patient inappropriately. Battery is the actual act of inappropriate touching. People who provide unpaid assistance to the injured in emergency situations are protected from assault and battery charges under the Good Samaritan Law.

## CONTRACT LAW IN DENTAL PRACTICE SITUATIONS

There is an expressed or an implied contract between the dentist and patient. The dental assistant or other personnel are the dentist's agents. The dentist is ultimately responsible for breach of contract under the Doctrine of Respondeat Superior. Nevertheless, the assistant's words or actions regarding care are legally binding upon the dentist. Breach of contract is failure to fulfill and complete the terms of the contract. There are **four situations where a contract can be legally abandoned**:

- The patient releases the dentist by failure to return for treatment; ideally, the patient sends the dentist a certified letter of discharge, but this is not required.
- The patient/guardian does not comply with specific instructions from the dentist regarding care.
- The patient no longer requires treatment.
- The dentist formally withdraws from the case by sending a certified letter to the patient explaining the situation, to preclude any charges of patient abandonment.

## THREATS OF MALPRACTICE

**Legal issues** related to dentistry include **threats of malpractice.** If a patient threatens malpractice, it's important to avoid arguing or making excuses. In order to prove malpractice, the patient must be able to show that he or she suffered an injury of some type as the result of dental care. The certified dental assistant should listen patiently and should carefully document any specific complaints that the patient makes, using quotations and including the date and time and any witnesses. If the patient is angry, sometimes simply being allowed to vent may solve the problem, but if the patient is in a public area, the certified dental assistant should suggest a more private area and should advise the patient to discuss the matter with the dentist. Because malpractice is a legal issue that is generally handled by attorneys, the practice may have an established protocol for dealing with complaints, and that protocol should be followed exactly.

## PATIENT'S RIGHT TO REFUSE RECOMMENDED TREATMENT

There are times when a patient will refuse to consent to recommended dental care. This may be routine procedures or complex surgical procedures. Even if a treatment is highly recommended or could prevent the patient from suffering serious consequences, the patient may still choose to refuse treatment.

For the patient to make an informed decision regarding their dental treatment, the treatment should be clearly communicated. The steps of the procedure should be explained, along with expected outcomes and the probability of a positive outcome. The risks of the procedure should be clearly explained, as well as the risks of potential complications if the patient does not want to have a procedure performed.

If a patient refuses treatment, it is important to clarify the reasons for making this decision. The decision may be financial and the office may be able to offer a reduced cost or payments may be set up to help with affordability. More education can be given if the patient is scared of the procedure and is worried about pain or other side effects from the procedure. Nonetheless, the patient has the right to refuse recommended care and the dental assistant should not carry out treatment without patient approval.

## RIGHTS OF PATIENTS IN DENTIST-PATIENT RELATIONSHIP

According to the **ADA's Dental Patient Rights and Responsibilities Statement**, patients should be given the following rights in the dental office:

- The right to choose their dentist and appointment time.
- The right to be informed of the dentist's training and education.
- The right to arrange to see their preferred dentist for each treatment (per state policy).

- The right to be granted the time to ask questions and get answers regarding dental treatment and conditions.
- The right to be informed of the dentist's opinion in terms of optimal treatment, and to be informed of alternative options.
- The right to informed consent, with a detailed explanation of the purpose, likely results, alternatives, and possible risks involved with dental procedures.
- The right to be informed of continuing health care needs.
- The right to know the cost of treatment prior to the procedure.
- The right to refuse treatment.
- The right to make reasonable arrangements for emergent dental care.
- The right to receive respectful and confidential treatment by the dental team.
- The right to expect proper infection control measures to be utilized by the dental team.
- The right to inquire about processes for mediating disputes about treatment.

## PATHWAYS TO TAKING THE CERTIFIED DENTAL ASSISTANT EXAMINATION

There are three possible pathways a candidate can take to the Certified Dental Assistant (CDA) examination or the General Chairside (GC) component through DANB. All three pathways require the candidate to have earned DANB-accepted cardiopulmonary resuscitation (CPR) certification within the previous two years. The candidate can write the Radiation Health & Safety (RHS) and Infection Control (ICE) examinations without the following prerequisites:

- **Pathway I** requires graduation from an ADA-accredited program for dental assisting or hygiene.
- **Pathway II** requires a high school diploma, or equivalency, with 3,500 hours of documented work experience as a dental assistant, either full-time over two years, or a combination of full and/or part-time within four years.
- **Pathway III** means the candidate is currently or was previously a DANB CDA or has a dental degree (DDS, DMD or foreign).

## GENERAL CERTIFICATION REQUIREMENTS FOR DENTAL AND ORTHODONTIC ASSISTANTS

Not all states require national certification for dental or orthodontic assistants. The Dental Assisting National Board, Inc. (DANB) offers written or computerized examinations for national certification. The CDA or Certified Dental Assistant exam has three parts: General Chairside (GC), Radiation Health & Safety (RHS) and Infection Control (ICE). The COA or Certified Orthodontic Assistant exam has two parts: Orthodontic Assisting (OA) and the ICE, both of which must be passed within a five-year period. Yearly continuing education and renewal is required for maintenance. Many states require DANB or some other type of licensure for performance of certain functions. DANB also administers examinations for the Certified Dental Practice Management Administrator (CDPMA) exam.

# Maintaining and Controlling Supplies and Equipment

## SUPPLY AND INVENTORY CONTROL

The aim of **supply and inventory control** is to have adequate supplies on hand but to avoid oversupplies with a goal of 8 to 12 inventory turns per year with shelf lives no longer than 3 months for expendable (consumable) supplies. For that reason, expiration dates must be considered when managing inventory because outdated supplies, including medications, must be disposed of. New supplies should be placed behind those already stocked so that the supplies are rotated according to expiration date. Backorders can pose a problem if orders are placed at the last minute, resulting in the need to order from different suppliers or to substitute other supplies. A record of backorders should be maintained to determine if there are patterns in the types of backorders and the timing of backorders. Critical supplies should be maintained at a higher inventory level than those used less frequently. All shipments received should be checked for completeness and inspected for damage. The projected life expectancy of nonexpendable supplies (equipment) should be factored into purchases.

## REORDERING SUPPLIES

Two common methods of **reordering supplies** are the red flag reorder tag system and the electronic bar code system. In the red flag reorder tag system, a tag is affixed to an item in inventory at the previously identified reorder point. At minimum, the name of the supply is on the tag. When the product reaches the reorder point, the tag is removed and put in a specified area for reordering. Every type of supply has an index card with information needed for ordering. The tag is attached to the upper-right corner when the item should be ordered, the left-hand corner after ordering, and removed upon receipt. New inventory is placed in the back of the pile and the red tag reaffixed at the new reorder point. With an electronic bar code system, supplies that must be reordered are identified by a specific bar code that is kept in a book. The assistant sweeps a bar code wand over the appropriate code, inputs the number of items needed, and the order is sent directly to the supplier via computer.

## INVENTORY SUPPLIES

The dental assistant usually orders supplies because he/she has clinical knowledge and surveys the stock daily. Supplies are either **expendable** (disposable and quickly consumed) or **non-expendable** (enduring and purchased rarely). The assistant must consider:

- Shelf life (expiry date) and rate of use.
- Storage space and special requirements (e.g., ice, dark, dry, fume hood).
- Single item price, unit price for grouped items, and bulk price (cut-rate price for ordering a minimum number of units), and price break (the smallest number of units needed to obtain a bulk price).
- Lead time between ordering and delivery, which determines the reorder point at which a supply needs to be bought in order to ensure continued availability.

## PROPER STORAGE METHODS

**Sterile supplies** should be placed in a storage area maintained at 65 to 72 °F with 35 to 50% humidity and at least 10 air exchanges (positive to adjacent areas) per hour. Supplies should be placed on shelves or in cabinets or carts and be at least 8 inches above the floor, 18 inches from the ceiling, and 2 inches from outside walls, using care not to crush or puncture the outside wrappings. Sterile supplies should never be stored under sinks or where they may be exposed to liquid (such as near water or sewer pipes).

**Nitrous oxide (NO₂) and oxygen (O₂) cylinders** should be safely secured so that they cannot fall in a non-public storage area and away from all grease and oil because of the potential for explosion. In the United States, $NO_2$ cylinders are blue and $O_2$ tanks green. Tanks should be protected against temperature extremes. The storage area should contain a sign indicating that the gases are present and no smoking or open flames are allowed.

## GENERAL DENTAL INSTRUMENT CARE

Most dental instruments are made of stainless steel, or occasionally aluminum or high-tech resins. Clean them promptly after use by immersion in an ultrasonic bath or instrument washer. Instruments that cannot be cleaned right away should be presoaked temporarily. Separate the blades of all instruments. Ultrasonic solution should cover all the instrument parts. Instruments that have hinges (e.g., scissors and forceps) should be sanitized first and later sterilized in the open position. Remove instruments from the ultrasonic bath, hold them under running water, dry, and then sterilize them. Sterilization techniques include liquid chemical disinfectants, ethylene oxide, hot glass bead, dry heat, chemical vapor, and steam autoclave sterilization. Dry the instruments well prior to storage. Some instruments have different or additional maintenance requirements. For example, burrs and handpieces must be scrubbed first, and since handpieces are attached to a power source via tubing, they need initial flushing and lubrication.

## ROTARY INSTRUMENTS, TRAPS, AND SUCTION LINES

Described below are ways to maintain these dental equipment/instruments:

- **Rotary instruments:** The central console and hand piece should be wiped down with a soft cloth dampened with disinfectant. The hand piece cartridge nut, heat shield, heat pluggers/thermal response tips, and entire motor should be autoclaved. The cartridges are for single patient use and should be cleaned or sterilized after use.
- **Traps:** Chemical cleansing compounds are usually used to clean the traps to remove organic materials. There are microbiology-based cleaning bacteria, also, that provide a less caustic and more natural way to clean debris from traps. These cleaning products contain bacteria that actually breakdown the organic matter. Cleaning should be done according to the guidelines provided by the manufacturer of the evacuation system.
- **Suction lines:** Should be disinfected daily with a compound that is compatible with the evacuation system. Buildup of tissue and debris within the lines can lead to low pressure through the lines. If patients close their mouths tightly around the suction tip, it can create a backflow and any debris in the lines can be recirculated back to the patient's mouth.

## DENTAL LABORATORY EQUIPMENT THAT MUST BE MAINTAINED

All dental laboratory equipment must **be decontaminated and maintained** in safe condition or retired. A dental laboratory technician may perform maintenance of complex equipment at the office, but often it is the dental assistant's responsibility. Much of the equipment is for taking impressions, creating trays, or making casts. These include the gypsum vibrator, extruder guns, lathes, model trimmer, hydrocolloid conditioning unit, soldering and welding equipment, and vacuum former. Most of these ship with explicit manufacturer-provided instructions, or obtain a copy from the sales person. Instruments that must be cleaned between uses and checked for wear include spatulas, laboratory knives, reusable impression trays, flexible rubber bowls, and measuring devices.

## RECEIPT AND STORAGE OF SUPPLIES

Examine all supplies received for damage. Look for inaccuracies and backorders on the packing slip enclosed with the shipment. If there is any damage or discrepancies, contact the supplier. Regular suppliers do not enclose a statement of payment due; it is sent separately to the practice on a monthly basis. A backorder is an item not immediately available; the supplier gives an estimated shipment date. If any units are returned, the supplier should issue the practice a credit slip, indicating there will be no charge. After receipt, the dental assistant should transfer the supplies to a well-organized storage area. Place older items in front to be utilized first. In a dental office, certain items are stored in a refrigerator or in a dark, dry spot. Controlled substances must be in a locked cabinet. Remember that thieves target dental offices for gold and addicts look for narcotics and syringes.

# Four-Handed Chairside Dentistry

## Four-Handed Dentistry Techniques

### EQUIPMENT IN DENTAL TREATMENT AREA

Order the **following equipment for the treatment room**:

- A comfortable, supportive dental chair with arm supports and an adjustable headrest and controls. The chair must accommodate upright, supine and sub supine positions.
- Ergonomic chairs or stools for both operator and assistant. The operator's (dentist's) chair should have 5 castors, an adjustable seat and back, and a broad base. The assistant needs a chair with a foot bar for support.
- Track-mounted, iridescent operating light to illuminate the oral cavity.
- An air-water syringe to provide streams of water and/or air.
- An oral evacuation system that includes a saliva ejector and a high velocity evacuation (HVE) device.
- A curing light, an electronically-controlled blue light-emitting wand that polymerizes resins and composites.
- Various handpieces operated by a foot-controlled rheostat or resistor attached to the dental unit.
- If restorations are performed, use an amalgamator to make the materials.

### TREATMENT ROOM PREPARATION

The dental assistant is responsible for **preparing the treatment room** between patients. This includes cleaning, disinfecting, and placing barriers on all areas (including charts) that may be touched. The Infection Control (ICE) exam covers appropriate procedures. The assistant pulls the rheostat, chairs, and mobile carts out of the patient's pathway, and lifts up the dental light. The dental chair should be about 15 to 18 inches above the floor, with the arm positioned for patient access. The dental assistant reviews the chart and sets out any needed radiographs, trays or lab work.

### GREETING AND PREPARING THE DENTAL PATIENT FOR TREATMENT

After preparing the treatment room, the assistant then **greets the patient** by name in the reception area and escorts him/her to the treatment room. The assistant illustrates where to put personal items. The assistant offers mouthwash, tissues for lipstick removal, a lip lubricant, and a drink of water to the patient and then seats him/her in the dental chair. The dental assistant puts the bib apron on the patient and gives him/her safety glasses to wear. The assistant asks about changes in the medical history, and inquires whether the patient has any questions. The assistant places the most recent radiographs on the view box. The assistant positions the patient supine for treatment, with the headrest supporting the head. The assistant adjusts the rheostat, operator's chair, assistant's stool, and lamp. The assistant dons a mask and protective eyewear. After washing his or her hands, the assistant dons gloves, then sets up trays, saliva ejector, air-water syringe, evacuator, and handpieces.

### DENTAL UNIT AND DENTAL HANDPIECES

The **dental unit** is the center from which **dental handpieces** and other essential equipment, such as the oral evacuator and air-water syringe, are controlled. The unit is set up to deliver instruments to the dentist from the rear, on the side of the dentist, or transthorax (over the patient's chest).

There are at least two high-speed and one slow speed handpiece and an air-water syringe connected to the unit. Slow-speed handpieces are straight and are used for decay removal, fine finishing, and polishing. Accessories are attached to the end, depending on the intended use. Slightly bent contra-angle attachments hold either friction-grip (FG) or latch-type (RA) burrs. The prophylaxis angle holds the polishing cup or brush. Low-torque, high-speed handpieces have curved ends. They are used with hard carbon steel burrs or diamond stones to remove the greater part of tooth structure for restoration before refinement. The friction generated necessitates use of a cooling water spray. The assistant is responsible for evacuation.

## FOUR-HANDED DENTISTRY TECHNIQUE

The **four-handed dentistry technique** is one in which the dental assistant and operator (dentist) are seated on either side of the patient and work together as a team. Using the clock face as a frame of reference, the patient's head is at 12. If, for example, a right-handed operator is on the right side and the dental assistant opposite, the operator zone is between 8 and 11 and the assistant's zone between 2 and 4. A left-handed operator may have a slightly wider operator zone, and the operator may sit at position 12 for some procedures. The transfer zone where instruments are passed (under chin, over chest) and received is from 4 to 8. The static zone is from 11 to 2. The dental assistant should sit close to and facing the patient at a level about 6 inches above the dentist. During instrument transfer, the assistant should use minimal motions, and the operator should keep eyes on the treatment site.

## SINGLE-HANDED AND TWO-HANDED INSTRUMENT TRANSFER TECHNIQUES

The assistant should transfer instruments within the transfer zone over the patient's chest. Both operator and assistant wear gloves. Transfer instruments with minimal motion. Keep the working end pointed toward the tooth being repaired. Keep the handle available for the dentist to grasp.

- In the **single-handed transfer technique**, the clinical assistant picks up the instrument from the tray, using the thumb and first two fingers of the left hand. The assistant holds the handle end or the side not required and places it into the transfer zone, near the implement in use. Exchange the instruments by using the last two fingers of the left hand for retrieval of the used one. Fold the used instrument into the palm. Simultaneously, put the new tool into the operator's fingers. Return the used instrument to its correct position in the setup tray.
- In the **two-handed technique**, grip the new instrument similarly in the right hand. Recover the used implement with the left hand and return it to the tray by releasing the palm grasp. Give the new instrument to the dentist with proper orientation of the working end.

## SITUATIONS REQUIRING UNIQUE INSTRUMENT TRANSFER TECHNIQUES

The operator uses the mouth mirror and explorer for examination at the beginning of the procedure. These are transferred from the assistant to dentist at the same time, using the two-handed technique. Most instruments are gripped by the dentist in a pen, palm, or palm-and-thumb grasp. The assistant holds pliers and forceps over their hinges and puts the handles directly into the dentist's palm or over his or her fingers. To transfer using cotton pliers, squeeze the beaks together to avoid dropping the cotton. Transfer dental materials much closer to the chin than instruments. The dental assistant can either give amalgam to the dentist or, if allowed by state law, directly insert it into the tooth. Transfer impression materials and cements delivered via syringes directly to the dentist, with the tip facing the arch where he/she is working. Convey cements and liners on mixing slabs, along with the applicator device. The assistant uses his or her right hand to hold the slab. The left hand wipes off any excess with gauze.

## GENERAL OPERATING ZONES IN TEAM DENTISTRY

Team or four-handed dentistry requires **four distinct zones** in the treatment area:

- A *static zone* right behind the patient, where the dental unit and a moveable cabinet are located.
- The *operator's zone* is the largest segment, to the left or right of the static zone, where the operator (dentist/hygienist/nurse) sits and moves around. Placement depends on whether the dentist is right-handed or left-handed.
- The *assistant's zone* is directly opposite the operator with the instrument cart and dental materials.
- A *transfer zone* next to the assistant is over the patient's chest, where assistant and operator exchange dental materials and instruments.

These four operating zones are often described in terms of a clock face with 12 divisions: The static zone occupies 2 portions; the operator occupies 5 portions; and the combined assistant and transfer zones making up the remainder (5 portions).

## PROPER SEATED POSITIONS FOR DENTAL OPERATOR AND ASSISTANT

The dental operator (dentist, hygienist, or nurse) sits with a straight back, feet planted on the floor, and knees slightly below hip level. Adjust the chair height level so the patient's mouth is level with the operator's elbows. The operator should be relaxed, with eyes directed downward toward the patient.

The assistant sits 4 to 5 inches higher than the operator to permit greater visibility and access. Sit up straight, with the abdominal bar or chair back in a supportive position. Place feet on the base platform, not the floor. Keep hips and thighs parallel to the floor, level with the patient's shoulders.

Dental operators experience shoulder, neck and back pain. Pain in the shoulder and neck is due to extended strain or flexion. Pain in the neck and back is due to prolonged extension or lifting of the arm. Low back pain is due to prolonged twisting. Carpal tunnel syndrome is a repetitive strain injury from prolonged wrist flexion and extension, as when keyboarding.

## MAINTAINING FIELD OF OPERATION USING IRRIGATION

The GCA is responsible for **irrigating** the dental operative site as necessary during a procedure. Irrigating the oral cavity when necessary allows small pieces of tooth material, blood, and debris to be washed loose so they can be removed via suction. This allows for a cleaner operative site that is easier to visualize.

The GCA can use a hand tool to perform irrigation, but additional irrigation is usually necessary to remove all of the material. Some dentists may not want to use the hand tool for irrigation during certain procedures. Frequently, the GCA will be responsible for operating the 3-way syringe which has a rotating tip to perform, irrigation, aspiration, or air to be applied to the operative site. Depending upon the manufacturer guidelines, the tip is usually removable for sterilization. The GCA may also use a syringe with normal saline or sterile water for irrigation. This is performed with a bulb-type or Luer syringe. Following irrigation, the fluid and debris is suctioned from the operative site.

## RETRACTORS AND MOUTH PROPS

**Retractors** redirect tissue, so the dentist sees clearly during procedures. Retractors are for oral surgery, but have other applications, too. There are tissue, cheek and lip, and tongue retractors.

Tissue retractors have small jagged edges on the working end to grasp tissue, and resemble forceps or cotton pliers. Cheek and lip retractors are large metal or plastic tools that fit into the mouth to pull the cheeks or lips outward, expanding the viewing region. Tongue retractors are spoon-shaped or lengthy blades that displace the tongue. Place tongue retractors between the rim of the tongue and the lingual surfaces of the teeth, or adapt them for cheek retraction by positioning them on the buccal mucosa. Hemostats and needle holders are forceps with jagged beaks and locking handles, usable for retraction. Insert mouth props when the patient's mouth must be open for a long period. They are stainless steel, silicone, plastic, or hard rubber, and come in various sizes. The locking Molt mouth gag is an example.

## ACCESS AND VISIBILITY IN FOUR-HANDED CHAIRSIDE DENTISTRY

The purpose of four-handed dentistry is not just to assist the dentist, but to also efficiently perform dental procedures in a way that will decrease physical stress. In order for true four-handed dentistry to be practiced, the clinical assistant should be in charge of the transfer of all instruments and all of the equipment should be within reach of the assistant. In order to have **optimal access and visibility**, the following criteria should be met:

- Excess motion should be minimized by using ergonomically-designed equipment.
- The patient should be in the supine position.
- The procedure team and patient should be situated comfortably in ergonomically-designed furniture.
- The personnel necessary for the procedure should be seated as close as possible to the patient the assistant should be sitting with his or her legs parallel to the patient chair.
- Use as few instruments as possible and have them arranged in order of use to increase efficiency.
- All materials used during a procedure should be placed in the appropriate area before the procedure to increase efficiency.

## MOUTH-RINSING METHODS

The dental assistant is responsible for both **mouth rinsing** and oral evacuation during dental procedures. Use either a saliva ejector or a more powerful high-volume oral evacuator (HVE). Perform limited-area rinsing often during pauses in the procedure to eliminate debris. Perform a complete mouth rinse at the end of the procedure. Grip the air-water syringe in the left hand and the saliva or HVE in the right hand. For a limited rinse, point the tip toward the desired area and direct air and water to the site. Suction out fluid and debris. Dry the site by compressing the air button. The patient should be facing the dental assistant during the final full-mouth rinse. Direct the HVE or saliva ejector tip into left part of the oral cavity (without touching tissues). Direct the air-water syringe first from right to left, along the maxillary arch, and then right to left along the mandibular arch. Place the suction tip in the back of the mouth to remove the fluid and extracted debris.

## ORAL EVACUATION METHODS

Moisture control and maintenance of a clinical field are paramount during dental procedures. A **saliva ejector** is a small flexible tube attached to a bulb, used for oral evacuation of minute quantities of saliva or water. A **high-volume oral evacuator (HVE)** is needed for large quantities of saliva and water, or for blood, pus, and vomitus. The HVE is essentially a vacuum with a sterile tip attached. Tips can be made of plastic or stainless steel. Tips are either straight or slightly angled, and the working end slants. Hold the evacuator with either a pen or thumb-to-nose grasp in the same hand as the dentist uses. Use the other hand to operate the air-water syringe or for instrument transfer. The patient's tongue and cheek must be isolated from the evacuation site with the HVE tip or the mouth mirror. There are several techniques for HVE tip placement, including on the lingual or buccal surfaces, slightly behind the prepped area, or on the opposite side of the tooth.

## PLACEMENT OF HIGH-VOLUME EVACUATOR IN POSTERIOR VERSUS ANTERIOR AREAS

When using an **HVE (high-volume oral evacuator) in posterior areas**, position the beveled edge of the tip as near to the tooth being prepared as possible, and parallel to either the buccal or lingual surface. The upper edge of the tip should reach a bit beyond the occlusal surface. Place a cotton roll under the tip for comfort when mandibular areas are being controlled. For anterior or front teeth, position the HVE tip parallel to the opposite surface and somewhat beyond the incisal edge of the tooth being prepared. Lingual and facial preparations require vacuum extraction from the facial and lingual sides, respectively.

## DRY ANGLES

**Dry angles** are triangular-shaped, absorbent pads that may be used during oral procedures in the back areas of either dental arch. Position the angles on top of the Stensen's duct, on the inside of the cheek, near the maxillary second molar. One type of salivary gland, the parotid gland, leads to the Stensen's duct. Therefore, the main purpose of dry angles is to obstruct the saliva flow into the area. The pads also preserve the oral tissues. Replace dry angles that become saturated with saliva. Moisten them further with the air-water syringe before removal.

## COTTON ROLLS

**Cotton rolls** isolate and control moisture in a working area during an oral procedure. For maxillary placement, the patient faces the assistant with his or her chin elevated. The assistant uses cotton pliers to grasp and convey the cotton roll to the mucobuccal fold nearest the working area of the patient's mouth. For mandibular placement, the patient faces the assistant with his or her chin lowered. The assistant picks up the cotton roll with the cotton pliers and transfers the roll to the corresponding mucobuccal fold. Place a second cotton roll on the floor of the mouth, between the operational field and the tongue. Ask the patient to raise his or her tongue to facilitate placement. Bend cotton rolls used in anterior regions before positioning. Take rolls out before the final full-mouth rinse, using cotton pliers. Very dry rolls can stick to the oral mucosa causing tissue damage. If a roll sticks, moisten it with water from the air-water syringe before removal.

# Dental and Intraoral Procedures

## BITING FORCES

Anything that exerts a push or pull on an object is a **force**. The object resists the force, causing stress. Significant stress causes a strain or alteration in the object. **Three forms of stress and strain** can occur:

- *Tensile force*, or outward stretching and pulling, potentially causing elongation. Elastic bands used in orthodontics can cause tensile stress and strain.
- *Compressive force* or pushing together, which occurs during chewing or biting.
- *Shearing* or portions sliding across one another from side to side, such as when people grind their teeth (bruxism). It is important to select dental materials that can withstand tensile and compressive forces, properties known as ductility and malleability, respectively.

All of these types of stress and strain apply to dentistry; consider them when selecting dental materials, because biting forces are significant. People bite down on molars with forces in the range of 130 to 170 pounds, and about a quarter of that is on incisors.

## HAND CUTTING INSTRUMENTS

Prior to use of handpieces, **hand cutting instruments** were used to prepare cavities. Now, hand instruments are for fine detailing. They consist of a central shaft or handle connected to shanks on one or both ends, attached to a bevel and some type of working end, usually a blade and cutting edge. The hand instrument is described in terms of its shank angles (e.g., straight, slightly curved or Wedelstaedt, monangle, binangle, and triple angle) and the class of cutting edge. There are five common classes of cutting edge: Hatchet, chisel, hoe, margin trimmer, and angle former. Both hatchets and hoes plane cavity walls and floors. The dentist uses a pulling motion. Hatchets and angle formers hone angles. Chisels are used with a pulling motion to plane enamel margins and to trim margins on front teeth. Special gingival angle formers (gingival margin trimmers), which have curved working ends, shape the cervical cavosurface margin in amalgam and inlay restorations. Excavators have more rounded blades to extract decay and debris.

## BURRS USED WITH SLOW-SPEED HANDPIECES

A **burr** is a tool attached to the end of a handpiece to remove rough edges of tooth structure. They are composed of stainless steel, or carbide metal, or diamond chips. The shanks to which the head (working end) and neck are attached are either friction-grip (FG), latch-type (RA), or straight handpiece (HP) types. There are a variety of types of **slow-speed burrs**, including:

- Acrylic burrs (used for acrylic-based dentures or orthodontic appliances).
- Straight HP finishing burrs (principally utilized for finishing gold, amalgam or composite restorations).
- Diamond stones (used for crown preparation).
- Green stones (for finishing gold, amalgam or composite restorations).
- Acrylic stones (again for acrylic dentures and orthodontic appliances).
- A mandrel or shaft can be connected to the handpiece and attached to sandpaper or abrasive discs with diamond or carborundum grit for finishing functions, or a bristle brush for tooth polishing.

## BURRS USED WITH HIGH-SPEED HANDPIECES

**High-speed handpieces** are principally used to remove undesired tooth structure swiftly, before finishing procedures. Therefore, burrs used with high-speed handpieces are made of carbon steel or diamond stones. Caries removal requires either round burrs or inverted cones. Round burrs open the pulp chamber for a root canal. Inverted cones are used for cavity preparation. Fissure burrs have flat ends and regularly spaced lines around the shaft. The straight fissure burrs, either plain cut or crosscut, make the initial opening into a tooth for smoothing the walls of a cavity or for axial retention grooves. The tapered versions are for inlay preparations or to open the pulp chamber for a root canal. Finishing burrs can be round, oval, pear or flame shaped. They are for finer aspects of amalgam or composite restorations. Wheel burrs form retentions. End cutting burrs form the shoulder for crowns. Burrs are numbered to reflect their shape, size and differences.

## BLACK'S FORMULA

G. V. Black invented a formula to describe hand cutting instruments in terms of the size of the blade and its angle relative to the shaft. There are two different formulae, a 3-number and a 4-number. The **Black's Three Number Formula** describes chisels, hatchets, and hoes. It consists of the first number for the width of the blade in tenths of a millimeter, the second number for the blade's length in millimeters, and the third number for the angle between the blade and the long axis of the shaft in degrees centigrade (parts per hundred of a complete circle). Thus, a blade designated as (18 8 15) is 1.8 mm wide, 8 mm long, and at an angle of 15/100 of a circle to the handle. The Black's Four Number Formula describes angle formers and gingival margin trimmers. Its first, third, and fourth number correspond to the same descriptions as the first, second and third numbers in the Three Number Formula. The fourth number represents the angle of the cutting edge relative to the handle.

## NON-CUTTING HAND INSTRUMENTS USED FOR BASIC EXAMINATION

Hand instruments not used for cutting fall into two classifications: Those used for basic examinations and those used to finish amalgam and composite restorative materials. **Non-cutting instruments** have configurations similar to cutting ones (handle, shank, and working end). **Basic examination implements** include mouth mirrors, explorers, cotton pliers, and periodontal probes. Categories of mouth mirrors include plane or regular with silver coatings on the glass back, front surface mirrors with rhodium on the front of the glass, and concave surface mirrors for magnification. The working end(s) of explorers are thin for probing; common configurations are the pigtail and shepherd's hook. Cotton pliers, which resemble large tweezers, transfer cotton rolls and other materials. Periodontal probes have round or blunt working ends and gauge the depth of the gingival sulcus.

## NON-CUTTING HAND INSTRUMENTS USED FOR FINISHING OF RESTORATIVE MATERIALS

**Non-cutting hand instruments** that are used for **finishing restorative materials** include filling instruments, amalgam carriers, amalgam condensers, carvers, burnishers, files, and finishing knives. Most have the same basic configuration of handle, shank and working end. Filling instruments, which put restorative materials and cement bases into the cavity preparation, are thermoplastic or anodized aluminum. Hand amalgam condensers (pluggers) press amalgam into the cavity preparation; there are also mechanical vibrating versions. Carvers are designed with working ends that can get rid of excess restorative agents or carve tooth anatomy; they are generally used on crowns, inlays and onlays. Burnishers smooth coarse margins or shape matrix bands. Both files and finishing knives, which have sharper ends, trim excess filling materials. Amalgam carriers load and place the amalgam; there are amalgam guns for composites, glass ionomers and alloys.

## MISCELLANEOUS HAND INSTRUMENTS FOR RESTORATIONS

**Miscellaneous hand implements** for restorations include spatulas, articulating forceps, and scissors. The commonly used spatulas are stainless steel cement spatulas for mixing cements and

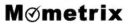

other materials, plastic for mixing composite resins, and larger general laboratory spatulas for blending impression materials or plaster. Articulating forceps grasp articulation paper (special heavy paper showing marks if contact is made) for checking occlusion after adding the restorative material. The type of scissor used most often for restorations is the crown and collar scissors (also called the bridge scissors), which have short straight or curved cutting blades. Scissors cut retraction cords and trim matrix bands.

## SCALERS, CURETTES, AND EXPLORERS

Scalers are hand-held instruments that remove undesirable substances from tooth surfaces. Most **scalers used for routine prophylaxis** are either sickle or curette scalers. Sickle scalers have long tapered tips with pointed toes. They are suitable for scaling under interproximal contact areas in the front of the mouth. Common sickle scalers include single-ended and double-ended straight sickles and a curved straight sickle (usually two or more curved cutting edges). Curette scalers can scale all tooth surfaces and are especially useful for removing subgingival calculus and root planing. They have rounded tips and backs and cutting edges. A universal curette is often employed for routine prophylaxis. It is straight and the entire edge is used to cut. Gracey curettes are designed to scale specific tooth surfaces or for root planing. They are curved at the end and only one side and the tip are used to cut. Gracey curettes are designated by their angles at either end, ranging from 1 for anterior teeth to 16 for posterior teeth surfaces. Dental explorers have very fine tips. They are used to check for calculus in subgingival regions during scaling.

## ULTRASONIC SCALER

Manual scalers have straight or curved sickles and pointed tips at each end; they are used most often to remove supragingival calculus. An alternative is the **ultrasonic scaler** (Cavitron), which removes heavy calculus and stain from tooth surfaces, cement, and bonding substances used in orthodontic work. An ultrasonic scaler uses high-frequency sound waves, which it translates into mechanical energy, in the form of high-speed vibrations at its tip. Water ejects at the tip to control heat buildup. The combination of vibrational energy and water facilitates thorough removal of debris. There are universal tips and narrower, slim line tips available. There are also sonic scalers, which are attached to the dental unit handpiece, and use air to remove calculus. Both have pen-like structures attached to their tips.

## SETTING UP THE ARMAMENTARIUM

**Armamentarium** refers to the supplies, equipment, and medicine used as part of medical/dental treatment. When utilizing the four-handed dentistry technique, the certified dental assistant should lay out the instruments and tools on the tray according to the order of use, which will vary depending on the type of treatment. The table with the instrument tray should be positioned so that the medical assistant can easily reach the instruments without changing position. Setups may vary according to preference.

| Procedure | Armamentarium |
|---|---|
| **Tooth desensitization** | Desensitizing agent (fluoride gel, sealant, dentin bonding agents, potassium nitrate corticosteroid), application brush. |
| **Tooth extraction** | Basic setup (mouth, mirror, cotton pliers, explorer). Anesthetic tray (Syringe, needle with recapping device, anesthetic agent, cotton-tip applicator, local topical anesthesia). Extraction forceps or dental elevator, curette (for scraping socket), suture materials (if indicated) with needle holder and suture scissors, hemostat, gauze. |
| **Tooth impaction** | Basic setup, Anesthetic tray, periosteal elevators, curettes, forceps, sutures, needles, surgical HVE tip, blade holder and appropriate blades, suture scissors, hemostats, lip retractors |

## CAVITY PREPARATION

**Cavity preparation** is the orderly cutting of tooth structure to remove any undesired portions, such decay, pits or fissures susceptible to caries, fractured tooth fragments, or enamel without underlying dentin support. The four steps of cavity preparation are:

1. Opening up the cavity with a burr.
2. Outlining.
3. Refining.
4. Finishing it with other instruments.

The dentist considers three and sometimes four factors when preparing a cavity. The first is the outline form or general shape of the preparation, which depends on the amount of decay, the material to be used, and how it can be retained. The resistance form is the internal contour of the cavity preparation. The dentist takes into account potential biting forces. The retention form is the internal profile of the cavity walls needed to keep the restoration in place, for example, using retention grooves or undercutting. There can also be a convenience form, which may be slightly larger than the outline form, to allow for use of instrumentation.

## PLACEMENT OF CAVITY LINERS, CAVITY VARNISH, AND CEMENT BASES

These procedures are executed by the dentist or the expanded-function dental assistant.

- **Cavity liners** include calcium hydroxide, glass ionomer or zinc oxide eugenol. Prepare as directed. Apply to the clean and dry cavity preparation. Place liner only into the deepest part of the preparation, using a ball attachment. Liners are either self-curing or light-cured for 10 to 20 seconds.
- **Cavity varnish seals dentin tubules**. Painted a thin layer over all exposed dentin with a cotton ball or pellet and sterile cotton pliers. Apply a second coat. Avoid contaminating the varnish.
- **Cement bases** are applied to the cleaned cavity preparation after a cavity liner and/or varnish. Mix the cement base materials as directed to a thick texture. Place onto the floor of the cavity preparation using a plastic filling instrument. Allow room for the restorative material.

## MEDICATION FOR CAVITY PREPARATIONS

The dentist cleans the cavity and usually medicates it prior to inserting the restoration. **Medication** ensures maintenance of healthy pulp because it:

- Seals dentin tubules.
- Calms pulpal irritation.
- Stimulates pulp healing.
- Provides a barrier between dentin and the restoration material for thermal insulation or to discharge fluoride into the area.

**Three substances** are used for medication: Thin, creamy cavity liners, like calcium hydroxide or glass ionomer; or cavity varnish; or cement bases, which include glass ionomer, zinc oxide and eugenol, and zinc phosphate. Suggested medication procedures depend on the restoration material and the depth of the cavity's preparation. For ideal depth cavity preparations, rinse the tooth and dry it with the air-water syringe.

## MEDICATION PROCEDURES AFTER CAVITY PREPARATIONS FOR AMALGAM OR COMPOSITES

Metal amalgam restorations require either two thin coats of cavity varnish or one of glass ionomer placed over the exposed dentin. Glass ionomer is recommended for composite or acrylic restorations. These are cavity liners. If the cavity preparation is of moderate depth, a cavity liner is also sufficient for amalgam restorations. Glass ionomer liners are suggested for composite restorations. Very deep cavity preparations require more extensive **medication techniques**. For amalgam restorations, usually the dentist applies calcium hydroxide to the deepest part then a cement base, and finally, two layers of cavity varnish. For composite restorations, an initial calcium hydroxide liner in the deepest portion should be followed by a glass ionomer base before the composite is added.

## AMALGAM

**Amalgam** is an alloy, a mixture of metals or metal and some nonmetallic material. Dental amalgam consists of silver, tin, copper and sometimes zinc which is then mixed with mercury. Unalloyed liquid mercury is a neurotoxin; treat it as a hazardous material. The way in which the dental alloy portion of the amalgam was prepared affects its properties, especially the relative concentration of components and the shape of copper particles. The major component (40% to 70%) of dental alloys is silver, which combines with the mercury to form a compound that eventually hardens. Tin, found in concentrations from about 22% to 37%, has a strong affinity for mercury and encourages the amalgamation. Copper increases the strength and hardness of the amalgam. Amalgams are usually defined as low copper (4% to 5%) or high copper (12% to 30 %), with the latter providing strength and corrosion resistance. Zinc may be added in small concentrations up to 1% to minimize the oxidation of the other metals.

Amalgam is **supplied** in color-coded capsules containing premeasured amounts of silver alloy powder and mercury. The color indicates whether the amount of material is appropriate for small cavity preparations (a single spill), or for larger cavities (double or triple spills). A metal or plastic pestle is provided for mixing the two ingredients when the capsule is opened. An amalgamator is an instrument for mixing and initiating the amalgamation (chemical reaction) between alloy and mercury. The success of this mixing procedure, also called trituration, depends on mixing time, speed of mixing, and force applied. Larger amounts must be mixed longer. The dental assistant prepares the capsule (twist-off cap, squeezing, or using an activator), puts it into the amalgamator, mixes it as determined, and after removal empties it into a container (Dappen dish or amalgam well).

## SPECIAL INSTRUMENTS

**Amalgam carriers** hold the amalgam and its pistons push amalgam into the site. Amalgam condensers are hand instruments with flat working ends that push the amalgam against surfaces of the cavity preparation. There are also automatic versions. Matrix bans are strips of thin stainless steel, used to fashion an outline around a prepared tooth. They are only necessary for restorations where tooth structure is lacking (class II, III and VI). The dentist uses the matrix band in parts to support condensation (pressing the amalgam into place). The matrix band is removed at the end of the restoration. A matrix retainer holds the two ends of the matrix band in place. A contouring plier shapes the matrix band. Interproximal wedges are three-sided wooden or plastic sticks that fit between the teeth after matrix band placement. Wedges prevent amalgam leakage into the interproximal space and keep adjacent teeth slightly apart. One wedge is needed for class II and III restorations. Two wedges are necessary for class IV and larger.

## TOFFLEMIRE MATRIX

The **Tofflemire matrix assembly** is the most widely-used matrix retainer for amalgam restorations. The central frame is connected at one end to a clamp-like vise. The vise has a diagonal slot through it, to grip the ends of the matrix band. Guide slots orient the matrix band loop in the correct direction. A screw-like spindle is connected to the vise and fixes the bands in place. At the opposite end is the outer adjustment knob, which is used to tighten the spindle alongside the band. Internal to that is an inner knob, which slides, and can be used for adjustment. Tofflemire setups are viewed from a gingival or an occlusal aspect, meaning the diagonal and guide slots are or are not visible respectively.

## PREPARE THE TOFFLEMIRE RETAINER AND MATRIX BAND FOR USE

When preparing the Tofflemire retainer and matrix band, hold the **Tofflemire assembly** in the left hand in a gingival aspect (slots toward the dental assistant or operator). Turn the outer knob clockwise until the spindle can be seen in the diagonal slot of the vise. Turn the inner knob until the vise is about 3/16 inch from the guide slots. Turn the outer knob counterclockwise, so the spindle is not visible in the diagonal slot. The dental assistant takes a matrix band, forming it first into a "smile" and then a loop. The occlusal edge makes the outer edge of the "smile." Insert the ends of the matrix band into the diagonal slot (occlusal edge on the bottom), while simultaneously threading the area closer to the loop into the guide slots. If the matrix band is for a tooth in the lower left or upper right quadrants, position the loop above the retainer. If the band is to for a tooth in the lower right or upper left quadrant, face the loop downward. Secure the band by turning the outer knob clockwise. Adjust the loop size with the inner knob. The shape can be rounded by using the handle of a mouth mirror.

## PLACEMENT AND REMOVAL DURING AMALGAM RESTORATIONS

**Place** the Tofflemire matrix over the prepared tooth. The correct placement is with the smaller edge of the band toward the gums, the diagonal slot toward the gingiva, and the apparatus parallel to the buccal surface. Push the band loop through the interproximal surface. Center it on the buccal surface of the tooth. Tighten the using the inner knob of the Tofflemire apparatus. Check the margins between the matrix band and cavity preparation to ensure that the band is not too tight or loose; they should be approximately 1.0 to 1.5 mm at the gingival edge and a maximum of 2 mm at the occlusal edge. Use a ball burnisher to contour the band, so there is contact with contiguous teeth. Place interproximal wedges at the gingival margins. Check with an explorer to ensure there are no gaps. After the dentist performs the restoration, remove the wedge(s) with cotton pliers or a hemostat. Loosen the retainer with the outer knob. Lift it off. Remove the matrix band with cotton pliers.

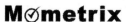

## APPARATUSES OTHER THAN TOFFLEMIRE MATRIX USED FOR RETAINING TEETH DURING RESTORATIONS

The main apparatuses other than the Tofflemire are the AutoMatrix, the plastic strip matrix, and sectional matrix systems.

- The **AutoMatrix** apparatus is convenient because it does not use a retainer. It comes with several sizes of conical bands that have tightening coils on the exterior for adjustment.
- **Plastic strip matrix systems** use thin, transparent strips, which are placed between the teeth, then around the preparation, and secured with a wedge. Secure the strip further after the restorative materials (not amalgam) are placed by pulling tightly and holding on or using a clip retainer. Plastic strips allow polymerizing light through. A variation is a crown matrix form, used for crowns on front teeth.
- **Sectional matrix systems** are comprised of relatively thick, contoured, oval matrix bands and rings to hold them. A discrete matrix band/ring pair is used for each tooth surface. Forceps are provided to open the rings. Wedges are put in between placement of the bands to position the rings. For pediatric patients, brass straight or curved T-bands or spot-welded matrix bands may be used.

## PIN-RETAINED AMALGAM RESTORATIONS

**Pin-retained amalgam restorations** may be used for teeth with extensive damage. After the cavity has been prepared, the dentist makes starter holes where needed. The dentist drills further between the pulp and external part of the root, using a unique twist drill. The dentist screws threaded pins into the holes with an autoclutch handpiece or a tiny hand wrench. Then the matrix band and retainer are positioned. The amalgam is added and condensed around the retention pins. The band is removed after hardening. Carving and finishing are performed as usual. Retention pins can also be used to make a central amalgam core, over which a cast gold crown is placed.

## CLASS II AMALGAM RESTORATION

**Class II amalgam restoration** assumes an expanded role for the dental assistant, working in conjunction with the dentist. Dry the injection site. Apply topical anesthetic. Convey the mirror, explorer, gauze, and a syringe filled with local anesthetic. The dentist injects the anesthetic. The assistant rinses and evacuates. Help the dentist as needed with placement of a rubber dam. Transfer the high-speed handpiece with burr and the mouth mirror to the dentist for inserting the amalgam restoration. Retract the cheek and tongue. Keep the mirror clear with the air-water syringe. Evacuate as needed with the HVE. Transmit and receive instruments, as requested. After the preparation, clean the tooth with a cotton pellet (rinsed and dried). Prepare and transfer to the dentist on cue the cavity liner, the cavity varnish, and the base. If light curing is required, direct the light tip.

After preparing the **Class II amalgam** restoration, assemble the matrix retainer and band apparatus. Hand it to the dentist in the correct orientation for placement. Transfer a wedge with cotton pliers or a hemostat. When the dentist indicates readiness, prepare the amalgam and activate it (twisting, squeezing, or putting in an activator). Mix in the amalgamator. Place the mixed amalgam into an amalgam well or Dappen dish. Load it into the amalgam carrier. Alternate placement of amalgam into the cavity preparation with packing with a condenser, until the cavity is filled. Amalgam may be placed by the dentist or assistant, but the condensing is a function of the dentist alone. When the filling is complete, the assistant transfers an explorer to the dentist for releasing amalgam from the matrix bind, cleans up amalgam fragments and puts them in a sealed container, and then hands carving, finishing, and band removal instruments as requested, while evacuating with the HVE. Remove the rubber dam. Dry the site. Use articulation paper to check

93

occlusion before cleaning off the patient. Instruct the patient not to chew on the filled side for several hours.

## PRECAUTIONS RELATED TO MERCURY USE

**Mercury** is toxic to nerves. It is liquid at room temperature and can vaporize. Take precautions at every step where exposure might occur. Follow the American Dental Association's guidelines for mercury use in the dental office. Wear disposable gloves, a face mask, and goggles when working with amalgam. Use premeasured capsules. Triturate in an amalgamator with a protective cover. Do not touch mercury with bare skin. If contact occurs, wash with soap and water and rinse well. Handle mercury only over impermeable surfaces and away from heat sources, like autoclaves. Do not eat or drink near mercury. Use a water spray, high-volume evacuation, and a mask when cutting or polishing amalgam. Store amalgam scraps and mercury in capped, unbreakable jars before disposal as hazardous waste. Properly ventilate the office. Carpet is not appropriate flooring. Educate all staff about regular urinalyses and monitoring devices for mercury. A mercury spill kit must be available.

## COMPOSITE RESIN INLAYS

**Composite resin inlays** can be used for posterior restorations. Alternatives are gold or porcelain inlays. The dentist makes a replica or die of the tooth. The dental laboratory makes the inlay (which has high amounts of filler for strength). At the time of cementation, the dentist applies acid etchant to the prepared tooth, then bonding resin, followed by composite cement applied to the etched enamel and the interior of the inlay. The composite cement is a dual-cure bond agent because it has elements that need to be both light-cured and chemically-cured. The inlay is then placed into the cavity preparation, light cured, and attuned for margins and occlusion.

## INSTRUMENTS AND SUPPLIES FOR COMPOSITE RESTORATIONS

When restorations use **composite resins** or glass ionomers, a filling instrument places the material in the cavity preparation. Long plastic or Teflon-tipped filling instruments are available, but usually a pistol grip composite syringe (with inserted cartridge) is used, so injection can be slowly controlled. Clear matrix strips and clamp-like strip holders retain the material. Usually, a surgical scalpel finishes composite restorations. A slow-speed handpiece may be used with various finishing stones and/or sandpaper finishing discs attached via a mandrel for polishing and contouring. These instruments need a water-soluble lubricant to reduce heat and clogging. There are special polishing strips for interproximal areas inaccessible to discs; use them like dental floss. Crown restorations require celluloid crown forms filled with composite or acrylic, positioned over the prepared tooth until hardened, which are then discarded.

## DIRECT COMPOSITE VENEERS

**Veneers** are thin layers of tooth-colored materials that are bonded to the enamel surface of teeth for aesthetic reasons, such as reshaping, concealing stains, or disguising diastema (large spaces between adjacent teeth). Before any type of veneering, the assistant polishes the teeth with pumice and water. There are both direct and indirect resin veneers. Direct veneers are made in one sitting. The dentist etches the teeth with phosphoric acid gel and applies two coats of bonding resin to the etched portions. Matrix strips are used if needed. Then the dentist applies composite resin in layers, followed by light curing and shaping. Opaquers and body shades may also be used before contouring and finishing is performed.

## INDIRECT COMPOSITE VENEERS

For **indirect veneers**, the dentist takes an impression at the first sitting. The laboratory fabricates the veneers, which are bonded at another appointment. The dentist applies a priming agent followed by a bonding agent (without light curing) to the tooth side of the veneer. The dentist places the veneer and checks for the shade of bond agent until the correct one is found, then temporarily removes it. The assistant installs matrix strips on either side of the tooth to be veneered. The dentist acid etches it, applies bonding agent to both the etched enamel and the tooth side of the veneer, and sets the veneer. Excess bonding agent is removed by the dentist. The assistant light cures the site for about a minute before the dentist finishes it. Indirect composite veneers are not as strong as porcelain veneers.

## ETCHED PORCELAIN VENEERS

**Etched porcelain veneers** are very strong, and desirable for aesthetic restorations of upper teeth. The dentist:

- Uses a diamond stone with a high-speed handpiece to take off some of the labial enamel (a retraction cord may be used).
- Takes a polysiloxane or polyether impression, makes a stone model, and sends it to the dental ceramist, who makes the veneers and etches them with a silane primer to encourages bonding.
- Installs temporary composite veneers, which are removed at the next appointment.
- Wets the veneers and tests them for fit prior to cementation.
- Instructs the assistant to place a matrix strip between the teeth.
- Etches the enamel.
- Spreads a resin bonding agent over both etched enamel and the tooth side of the veneer.
- Applies a fine layer of the appropriate shade of resin bonding substance on the tooth side of the veneer.
- Instructs the assistant to light cure the site for about a minute.
- Finishes the site with suitable burrs and stones.

## CAST-GOLD RESTORATIONS

**Cast-gold restorations** include gold inlays, onlays, and bridges. All are made from gold alloys that have been melted and then cast and hardened into the needed shape. Gold alloys are readily melted, very strong to resist eating forces and edge fractures, non-corrosive, non-irritating, and non-allergenic. For gold inlays, the majority of the restoration is located within a tapered cavity in the tooth; these are appropriate for all cavity classes. Cast-gold onlays or crowns reach over the cusps of back teeth to ensure against fracture during mastication. Cast-gold crowns generally cover either three-quarters or the entire crown of the tooth. A three-quarter crown usually leaves the facial facet untouched for aesthetics. Cast-gold restorations always require two sittings: The first to prepare the tooth and take impressions before manufacture of the restoration in the laboratory (a temporary filling is inserted); and the second to fit and cement the restoration in place.

## CAST-GOLD INLAY RESTORATIONS

The dental assistant assists the dentist throughout with following procedural elements of **cast-gold inlay restoration**, and in some states is permitted to seat the retraction cord, make the final impression, and/or temporary filling. The dental team:

- Uses alginate to make an impression of the opposing teeth that will abut the finished inlay.
- Fits the bite registration onto an articulator, incorporating the opposing model impression, if possible.
- Applies topical anesthetic.
- Injects local anesthetic.

- Isolates the site with cotton rolls.
- Removes the rubber dam (if any).
- Retracts the gingiva.
- Prepares the cavity with smooth, slightly tapered walls for later insertion of the inlay.
- Uses hemostatic agents to stop bleeding.
- Removes the cord.
- Dries the cavity preparation is dried.
- Takes an impression using agar hydrocolloid, polyether or polyvinylsiloxane.
- Temporizes the cavity preparation with a temporary filling of ZOE (zinc oxide and eugenol) or plastic.

The following are the procedures for the cementation appointment for cast-gold inlays:

- Apply anesthetics.
- Isolate the site with cotton rolls.
- Carefully remove the temporary with a spoon evacuator or burr, cotton pellets, and the air-water syringe.
- Seat the inlay with a wooden peg, orangewood stick, or other seating device.
- Check where the inlay contacts proximal surfaces of adjoining teeth and the cervical areas; make necessary adjustments.
- Tell the patient to bite down on articulating paper.
- Look for marks indicating hyperocclusion or too high an inlay; grind down, if any.
- Polish the final form with abrasives, externally on the tooth, and then on the dental lathe.
- Disinfect the form.
- Wash, dry, and isolate the tooth for cementation.
- Pretreat the preparation with cavity varnish if using zinc phosphate cement; non-irritating polycarboxylate and glass ionomer cements is preferable.
- Blend the cement and layer it onto the prepared tooth surfaces.
- Position the inlay and seat it with finger pressure.
- Place a bite device over the inlay and instruct the patient to bite down until cement is set.
- Check and finish margins.

## PREPARATION APPOINTMENT FOR CAST-GOLD CROWN

Teeth for which **cast-gold crowns** are fabricated have more area removed than those receiving inlays. Prepare them with a high-speed handpiece and tapered fissure burrs or diamond stones. For full crowns, grind the complete occlusal surface to a clearance of three thicknesses of occlusal wax (28-gauge sheets of wax). Three-quarter crowns leave the facial aspect intact. The preparation appointment for cast-gold crowns includes the following procedures:

- Make a plaster model from an alginate impression.
- Make a plastic mold using a vacuum former with heating element (similar to making an acrylic resin custom tray).
- Fill the appropriate part of the mold with self-curing acrylics.
- Place this over the prepared tooth while the patient bites down during hardening.
- Remove the mold and separate it from the acrylic.
- Polish.
- Seat with temporary cement.

## ALL-CERAMIC RESTORATIONS

**All-ceramic restorations** are for occlusal and multiple-surface restorations. Usually, the laboratory makes them with porcelain or castable glass, called Dicor. They can be constructed chairside, using CEREC computerized design, which is expensive but only takes one sitting. The dentist prepares the cavity and makes a final impression, an opposing arch alginate impression, and a bite registration. The dental ceramist makes the restoration. The dentist installs a temporary acrylic filling. Prior to insertion at the next appointment (or same day for CEREC), the dentist etches the porcelain and applies silanizing agent for bonding. The dentist removes the temporary filing. The assistant cleans the tooth and positions matrix strips and wedges between proximal surface. The dentist etches the tooth, applies a bonding substance to the preparation, then dual-cure composite cement to both the preparation and the tooth side of the restoration. The dentist inserts the restoration and the assistant light cures it for about a minute on each surface. The dentist finishes it, tests the occlusion, and adjusts the restoration.

## CLASS II COMPOSITE RESTORATION
### ASSISTANT'S TASKS

- Rinses and dries the site.
- Applies topical anesthetic.
- Inserts a rubber dam to isolate the tooth.
- Keeps the area clear and evacuates it.
- Dries the preparation.
- Prepares the calcium hydroxide and/or glass ionomer base or liner for cavity medication and may light cure it.
- Rinses acid etchant.
- Mixes bonding agent, applies it, and light cures it.
- Holds the matrix tightly to maintain contours.
- Removes matrix strip, wedge, and dental dam.
- Examines the site, dries, and rinses it.

### DENTIST'S TASKS

- Injects local anesthetic.
- Selects the shade of composite material that matches the patient's teeth.
- Prepares the cavity.
- Applies acid etchant.
- Positions celluloid matrix strips, plastic wedges, and sometimes a primer.
- Adds composite incrementally with a filling instrument, followed by light curing or chemical self-curing.
- Tests the restoration with an explorer.
- Finishes restoration with a low-speed handpiece and abrasive attachments.

## CLASS IV AND V COMPOSITE RESTORATIONS

Composite restorations are called aesthetic because they are tooth-colored. Increasingly, composite restorations are being used for posterior teeth, even though they are grinding surfaces. Composites are appropriate for class III, IV, and V cavity preparations. **Class IV composite restorations differ from class III in these respects:**

- Pins are needed for retention in the cavity preparation.
- A cut-off portion of a celluloid crown form may be used to shape proximal and incisal portions.
- A celluloid crown form is used for composite insertion.

**Class V preparations** are usually easily filled with composite or glass ionomer, without matrix bands, and require minimal finishing. If the root surfaces are exposed, the tooth is conditioned with 10% polycyclic acid, the preparation is rinsed and dried, a calcium liner may be used, and then the composite or glass ionomer material is inserted.

## ARMAMENTARIUM FOR CROWN AND BRIDGE PREPARATION AND CEMENTATION

**Preparation**: Basic setup, anesthetic tray, periodontal probe, rubber dam setup, cords, bite block, temporary cement, crown and bridge bur block, viscostat, scissors, articulating paper, cord packer, cotton rolls, 2 x 2 gauze, triple tray X 3, impression material gun X 3, bite registration, light body, heavy body, bite registration tip, light body tip, heavy body tip, and tooth shade selector.

**Cementation**: Basic setup, crown and bridge preparation kit with regular, fine, and superfine diamond points, etchant, silane coupling agent, acetone, try-in paste, bonding agent, brush, resin luting agent, polymerization light, porcelain polishing kit.

## ARMAMENTARIUM FOR PLACEMENT OF STAINLESS-STEEL CROWNS

Armamentarium required for the placement of **stainless-steel crowns** include:

- *Topical and local anesthetic:* Medications, a long needle, a short needle, and syringes should be available.
- *Mouth mirror:* For visualization or the oral cavity and to reflect light.
- *Periodontal probe:* Used to measure the depth of the gingival sulcus and to evaluate for any recession of the gingival tissue.
- *Crown-contouring pliers:* Used for enhancing contours and accurately design the contacts and gingival margins for placement of the crown.
- *Crown crimping pliers:* Used to crimp the gingival margins of the crown for accurate fit and placement.
- *College pliers:* Serrated pliers with angled tips to allow better visualization of the procedure field.
- *Large spoon excavator:* Used to tooth excavating and remove of glass ionomer material.
- *Heatless stone:* Made of silicone carbide abrasive and used to grinding and shaping.
- *Burlew wheel:* A knife-edged polishing wheel used for finishing.
- *Appropriate size burrs:* Used for reshaping and finishing.
- *Stainless steel crown:* The prefabricated crown form that is fit to fit an individual tooth and cemented into place.

## DENTAL DAMS

**Dental dams** are commercially-available barriers used to isolate areas during oral procedures. The dam improves access for the dentist and assistant because it retracts the lips, tongue and gums. It also enhances visibility of the area by providing color contrast. Dams come in latex or latex-free materials in various sizes, colors and thicknesses. Dams are divided into sixths, with holes punched for placement in the upper or lower middle portion for maxillary or mandibular treatments, respectively. Employ dental dams for involved procedures requiring local anesthesia. The patient is less likely to accidentally inhale or swallow materials when a dental dam is used. A dental dam provides infection and moisture control. It inhibits contact with debris and dental materials. In some states, the dental assistant may legally place the dental dam.

## EQUIPMENT USED WITH DENTAL DAMS

The dental dam is held in a three-sided, plastic or metal dental dam frame for positioning. A dental dam napkin is a cotton sheet placed between the dam and patient to absorb moisture. A dental dam punch is a specialized type of hole-puncher to tailor holes in the dental dam exactly where the teeth need to be isolated. Punches come in five **ascending sizes**, and are specific to the type of tooth involved:

- No. 1 for mandibular incisors.
- No. 2 for maxillary incisors respectively.
- No. 3 for canines and premolars.
- No. 4 for molars and bridge abutments.
- No. 5, the largest, for the anchor tooth chosen to hold the dental dam clamp securely.

Dental dam clamps are made of stainless steel in the shape of the crown; they come in cervical, winged and wingless conformations, and have a bow, jaws and forceps holes. The dental dam forceps are for dam positioning and removal, adding lubricant, and a dental dam stamp. The latter is an ink-pad stamp made like a dental arch, which serves as a guide to indicate teeth to be punched out on the dam.

## PREPARATION FOR USE

**Before inserting a dental dam**, the dentist administers local anesthetic, with the help of the dental assistant, who must note any misaligned or malposed teeth at that time. If a tooth is abnormally positioned, punch holes in a corresponding spot in the dam. Note the width of the arch for possible accommodations. Apply lubricant to the patient's lip with a cotton roll or applicator. Use a mouth mirror and explorer to find a suitable location for dam placement. If there is any debris or plaque in the area, brush the teeth or apply coronal polish prior to dam positioning. Floss all regional contacts to avoid tearing the dam. Mark a dental dam stamp to identify the teeth for isolation in the correct arch. Using this template, punch the dental dam with the correct size of dam punch. Make a hole for the anchor and the tooth for isolation. Lubricate holes that stretch over tight contacts with water-soluble lubricant on the underside.

## PLACEMENT

When **placing a dental dam**, attach the correct clamp to both a floss safety line and a locked dental dam forceps. Fit the dam over the anchor tooth, initially over the lingual side. Widen the forceps, and place the dam over the buccal side. Place the previously punched dental dam over the clamp bow, using the index fingers to stretch it over the clamp and anchor tooth. Pull the safety line to the outside. Fasten the dam to the last tooth at the opposite end with floss or cord. Place the dental napkin between the outer parts of the dam and the patient's mouth. Affix the dental dam frame over the oral cavity to hold the dam in place. Isolate the other teeth through the punched holes and push them into place by using dental floss or tape. Dry the teeth with the air syringe. Seal all edges by tucking or inverting them into the sulcus of the gum with a tucking instrument, before performing the desired procedure.

## REMOVAL

The first step of **dental dam removal** is to stretch the dam material outward with the middle or index finger. Cut each interseptal dam. Remove the dam clamp with the dam forceps by placing them into the forceps holes and compressing the handles to open the jaws of the clamp. Rotate the clamp toward each side for easy removal. Remove the holder, dam material, and napkin. Examine the dam is examined to ensure no material is left interdentally. Floss the patient's teeth, if indicated. Knead the gum around the anchor tooth to improve circulation. Rinse the patient's mouth. Remove any remaining debris.

## TOPICAL FLUORIDE APPLICATION

**Topical fluoride application** in the dental office is usually done using 2% sodium fluoride, 8% stannous fluoride, or 1.23% acidulated phosphate fluoride (APF). Sodium fluoride preparations are stable, do not cause discoloration, and are gentle to tissues, but they must be applied weekly for four weeks each time. Stannous fluoride has many disadvantages, including instability, a caustic taste, and discoloration due to tin in the preparation. Thus, the APF preparations are used most often, as they are non-irritating, have a mild taste, do not cause discoloration, and need to be used only once or twice a year. Keep APF preparations in plastic containers to discourage acidification.

## PROCEDURES

The dental assistant performs **fluoride application** after a rubber cup polish. Never apply fluoride before placement of orthodontic bands or sealants, as it deters adhesion.

1. Don personal protective equipment (PPE).
2. Select fluoride trays that encompass all erupted teeth but do not extend beyond them.
3. Fill each tray one-third full with the fluoride gel or foam.
4. Dry the patient's teeth with the air syringe.
5. Position the trays in the patient's mouth and shift them up and down to distribute the fluoride preparation.
6. Keep the saliva ejector in the patient's mouth throughout the procedure to remove saliva and moisture. Instruct the patient to keep his or her mouth closed for the recommended time.
7. Remove the ejector trays. Evacuate the patient's mouth.
8. Advise the patient not to eat, drink, or rinse for 30 minutes following the application.
9. Using overgloves, chart the application and any consequences.
10. An alternative to foam or gel application is the use of a fluoride rinse after tooth brushing or a rubber cup polish.

## ARMAMENTARIUM FOR VARIOUS PROCEDURES

### TOOTH IMPLANT

Basic setup (mouth, mirror, cotton pliers, explorer). Anesthetic tray (Syringe, needle with recapping device, anesthetic agent, cotton-tip applicator, local topical anesthesia). IV solution, surgical HVE tip, sterile gauze and cotton pellets, irrigation syringe, sterile saline, low-speed handpiece, sterile template, sterile surgical drilling unit, scalpel, blades, periosteal elevator, rongeurs, surgical curette, tissue forceps, tissue scissors, cheek retractor, tongue retractor, hemostat, bite-block, oral rinse, Betadine, implant instrument kit, implant kit, suture setup.

### INCISION OR DRAINAGE

Basic setup, anesthetic tray, Bard Parker blade.

## PERIODONTAL SURGICAL DRESSING PLACEMENT AND REMOVAL

**Placement**: Basic setup, plastic instrument, gauze sponge, tongue depressors, mixing pad, periodontal dressing base/accelerator, cotton tip applicators, lubricant, saline, cold water, Gelfoam®.

**Removal**: Basic setup, suture scissors, plastic instrument, floss, saline solution, HVE tips

## DRY SOCKET

Basic setup, cotton balls, 2 x 2 gauze, topical anesthetic Eugenol, perioprobe, scissors.

## NON-REMOVABLE DENTURE PLACEMENT

**Armamentarium** required for **non-removable denture placement** includes the following:

- *Chlorhexidine gluconate*: Used as a one-minute pre-rinse to disinfect.
- *Surgery setup pack:* Necessary PPE, drapes, and covers.
- *Paper products*: Gauze, cotton rolls, cotton-tipped applicators.
- *Suction tips*: Sterilized tips for saliva ejector and suction.
- *Sterile titanium box:* To hold the implant if it needs to be removed and reinserted.
- *Antibiotic ointment*: Applied to the abutment threads to aid in healing.
- *Blood pressure cuff*: To monitor blood pressure during the procedure.
- *Basic setup*: 2 dental mirrors, 2 cotton pliers, a periodontal probe, a hemostat, suction holder, surgical scissors, retractors, and scalpels.
- *Local anesthetic*: Medications and syringes should be available.
- *Surgical handpiece and motor*: With a sterile saline pump with tubing for irrigation.
- *Drill kits*: Arranged in order of the recommended drilling sequence based upon the implant diameter.
- *Digital caliper*: Used to measure drill stop lengths.
- *X-ray sensor holder*: With a sterilized cover.
- *Tissue punch kit*: Provides access to the implant site with minimal trauma.
- *Backup dental implants*: In case one is dropped.
- *Healing abutments*: Various diameters.
- *Provisional crowns*: Including composite, primers, condensers, bonding instruments, and a dental curing light.

## OCCLUSAL EQUILIBRIUM/ADJUSTMENT

The purpose of **occlusal equilibration** is to equalize occlusal stress in order to create simultaneous occlusal contacts. The armamentarium required for this procedure are:

- *Chlorhexidine gluconate:* Used as a one-minute pre-rinse to disinfect.
- *Surgery setup pack:* Necessary PPE, drapes, and covers.
- *Paper products:* Gauze, cotton rolls, cotton-tipped applicators.
- *Suction tips:* Sterilized tips for saliva ejector and suction.
- *Basic setup:* 2 dental mirrors, 2 cotton pliers, a periodontal probe, a hemostat, suction holder, surgical scissors, retractors, and scalpels.
- *Blood pressure cuff:* To monitor blood pressure during the procedure.
- *Medications for sedation:* The procedure may be performed under sedation to make the patient more comfortable.
- *Small diamond wheel stone:* Used with a 12-sided football-shaped finishing burr for precise reshaping.

- *Marking ribbons:* Red and black marking ribbons are secured in Miller ribbon holders.
- *Topical fluoride:* May be administered to strengthen the enamel to better resist tooth decay and to decrease sensitivity.
- *Restorative dentistry materials:* Necessary if the patient will be receiving any onlays, fillings, or crowns following the procedure.

## ROOT PLANING AND CURETTAGE

Armamentarium for root planing includes the following:

- *Topical and local anesthetic*: Medications, a long needle, a short needle, and syringes should be available.
- *Mouth mirror*: For visualization or the oral cavity and to reflect light.
- *Periodontal probe*: Used to measure the depth of the gingival sulcus and to evaluate for any recession of the gingival tissue.
- *Scalars and curettes*: Used to remove calculus from the surface of the teeth. Curettes can also be used below the gum line, but scalars are only used above the gingival tissue.
- *Cavitron tips*: Uses high frequency sound waves to clean tartar from the surface of the teeth.

Armamentarium for curettage include the following:

- *Topical and local anesthetic*: Medications, a long needle, a short needle, and syringes should be available.
- *Mouth mirror*: For visualization or the oral cavity and to reflect light.
- *Periodontal probe*: Used to measure the depth of the gingival sulcus and to evaluate for any recession of the gingival tissue.
- *Gracey curettes*: Stainless steel instruments used to remove calculus. Designed with a cutting edge that can be used above and below the gingival tissue.

## GENERAL ORAL EXAM

The armamentarium required for the **general oral exam** include:

- *Setup pack:* Necessary PPE, drapes, and covers.
- *Paper products:* Gauze, cotton rolls, cotton-tipped applicators.
- *Mouth mirror:* For visualization or the oral cavity and to reflect light.
- *Explorer:* Used to examine tooth surfaces, evaluate root surfaces, remove cement, and to check fit margins.
- *Cotton pliers:* For placement and removal of small objects from the oral cavity.
- *Periodontal probe:* Used to measure the depth of the gingival sulcus and to evaluate for any recession of the gingival tissue.
- *Saliva ejector tip:* Uses low-volume evacuation to remove saliva to dry the procedure field.
- *Oral evacuator tip:* Uses high-volume evaluation to remove blood, saliva, and debris. This can help to remove microbes. May also be helpful with retraction to protect the tongue and cheek.
- *Light:* Used with a disposable mouthpiece to adequately illuminate the oral cavity, aspirate, protect the throat, and retrace the tongue and cheek all in one device.
- *Anesthetic syringe:* Aspiration is performed to check for blood drawn into the syringe before local anesthesia is delivered.
- *Intraligament syringe:* Used to inject anesthesia into the periodontal ligament space to supplement a nerve block.

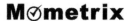

## ROUTINE PROPHYLAXIS
### ARMAMENTARIUM

**Dental prophylaxis** means preventing dental disease by identifying and removing plaque and debris from tooth surfaces. The armamentarium suggested for routine prophylaxis consists of various sickle scalers, a universal curette, an explorer, floss, a saliva ejector and HVE tip, a Dappen dish, disclosing solution, air and water syringe tips, cotton swabs, gauze sponges, prophy paste, and angle and ring holders. If root planing or smoothing is to be performed, include several Gracey curettes and a setup for local anesthesia, including the anesthetic.

### GENERAL PROCEDURES

Routine dental prophylaxis consists of an **assessment** and a **treatment phase**. During the assessment phase, the assistant applies disclosing agent to the patient's teeth to identify plaque accumulation. The treatment phase has four parts:

- Scaling or scraping off undesirable substances on the surfaces of teeth, such as hard calculus and softer plaque with various scalers, and using the explorer to check subgingival portions. The dental assistant aids the dentist by using the oral evacuator or gauze sponges. Root planing may be performed now or scheduled separately.
- Coronal polishing is performed with a dental handpiece and prophy paste or an air-powder abrasive polisher, to remove further plaque and stains and leave a smooth surface. Again, the assistant aids with evacuation.
- Flossing is performed to guarantee plaque removal between teeth.
- Fluoride treatment is an elective procedure.

## CORONAL POLISH

A **coronal polish** is a process by which soft deposits and extrinsic stains are removed from the clinical crown of teeth with abrasive material. The dental assistant will require a dental handpiece and a rubber cup for easiest application, but can substitute brushes, dental tape, or floss, if necessary. Perform coronal polishing after hard deposits are scaled away. The coronal polish is **performed for three main reasons**:

- It helps the patient maintain clean teeth and sustain good oral hygiene.
- The procedure enhances fluoride absorption and discourages buildup of new deposits.
- It prepares teeth for use of enamel sealant and for positioning of orthodontic brackets and bands.

In many states, the dental assistant or hygienist can legally perform a coronal polish. If the dentist delegates polishing to the dental assistant, the dental assistant should seat him/herself in the appropriate operator's position.

### ABRASIVE USE

**Abrasives** are rough, particulate materials that create friction to smooth out the tooth surface during coronal polishing. Abrasives come in powder or paste form, and usually contain water, a binder, and a humectant for water retention, coloring and flavoring. Available abrasive agents include fluoride pastes, flour of pumice, chalk, zirconium silicate, and tin oxide. The rate of abrasion for a particular type of abrasive is dependent upon the characteristics of the abrasive material, the speed of the handpiece, the pressure and amount applied, and the moisture level. Abrasion increases if the particles are sharp-edged, firmer, stronger, larger in size, or resist embedding in the tooth's surface.

## REMOVABLE AND NONREMOVABLE MATERIALS

A coronal polish can remove soft deposits and extrinsic stains. Calculus (hardened, calcified deposits) and intrinsic stains cannot be eliminated through coronal polishing. The dentist removes calculus is prior to the polish via scaling. Intrinsic stains are within the tooth structure and are usually permanent. For example, dental fluorosis, metal poisoning, tetracycline exposure in childhood or pulp damage cannot be removed by polishing. There are **five types of soft deposits removed by coronal polishing:**

- *Materia alba*, a less structured a precursor to plaque development, which contains microorganisms and leads to tooth decay, gingivitis and periodontal disease.
- *Plaque*, which contains microorganisms that damage teeth and gums.
- Food debris.
- *Pellicle*, a thin film containing saliva and sulcular fluid
- *Extrinsic stains* from endogenous sources can be removed by coronal polishing. For example, yellow or brown stains associated with poor dental hygiene and tobacco can be polished away.

## PROCEDURES USING A PROPHY BRUSH

**Prophy brushes** are soft, supple brushes made of nylon or natural bristles. Perform prophy brushing after the rubber cup polish. Attach one brush to a low-speed dental handpiece. Only polish the enamel surfaces of teeth. Do not allow the brush to contact the gums. Spread prophy paste over the brush. Start polishing the most posterior tooth. For the back teeth, the major objective is to polish the occlusal surfaces. For each posterior tooth, direct the brush from the central fossa first, toward the mesial buccal cusp tip, and then toward the distal buccal cusp. For the anterior teeth, position the brush in the lingual pit above the cingulum, and then toward the incisal edge during polishing. All lingual surfaces with pits or grooves should be polished similarly. At the end, rinse the patient's mouth and clear it of debris.

## PROCEDURES USING A RUBBER PROPHY CUP

Coronal polishing using a rubber prophy cup:

1. Apply disclosing agent to teeth with a cotton applicator for easier plaque recognition.
2. Ask the patient if he/she is allergic to latex rubber; if yes, choose a synthetic rubber cup.
3. Attach a prophy cup to a low-speed dental handpiece at an angle.
4. Place abrasive agent into the cup; if more than one type is required, use an individual cup for each.
5. Hold the handpiece with cup in a modified pen grasp.
6. Apply foot pressure on the rheostat to regulate speed.
7. Polish one quadrant at a time. Position the cup near the sulcus of the gum on the mesial or distal surface of a tooth. Employ gentle pressure to bend the cup. Work toward the occlusal or incisal edge. Lift the cup a little. Duplicate the procedure on the other side of the tooth.
8. Frequently rinse and remove debris during the procedure.
9. Repeat on the adjacent tooth, until all teeth are polished.
10. Reapply disclosing agent to check work.
11. Rinse.

## SUPPLEMENTAL EQUIPMENT

The dental assistant will also require a good dental light, cheek retractors, a mouth mirror, an air-water syringe, an evacuator, a saliva ejector, and wipes to polish teeth correctly. **Supplementary polishing aids** that might be useful during the final phase are dental tape and floss. One aid that is useful for patients with orthodontic work is a bridge threader, a plastic piece with a loop through which dental tape or floss is passed. A threader allows the assistant to work around orthodontic or other appliances. Various grit size abrasive polishing strips can be employed on enamel facades. Soft wood points can be used with abrasives. Small interproximal brushes can be utilized. The latter are especially useful for navigation around orthodontic appliances and other contact areas.

## DISCLOSING AGENTS

**Disclosing agents** are temporary coloring agents in chewable tablet and liquid forms, usually red. Disclosing agents adhere to plaque to help the assistant and patient identify it much more easily. The assistant uses agents to check coronal polishing technique. When the dental assistant or hygienist uses disclosing agent in the office, he/she should wear Personal Protective Equipment (PPEs). Spread petroleum jelly over the patient's lips and tooth-colored restorations. Decant agent into a Dappen dish. Paint the liquid agent onto the teeth with a cotton tip applicator or put it on the tongue to spread. Alternatively, ask the patient to chew a tablet and swirl it around in the mouth. Rinse and withdraw excess solution. Give the patient a hand mirror. The dental assistant may use a mouth mirror and air-water syringe. Chart the plaque present, using an overglove. Educate the patient education about oral hygiene. Disclosing agents encourage the patient to use good oral hygiene at home.

## POLISHING WITH DENTAL TAPE OR DENTAL FLOSS

After performing a coronal polish using a prophy cup and a prophy brush, polish them interproximally with **dental tape and floss**. Cut a 12- to 18-inch piece of dental tape. Apply abrasive to the interproximal contact places between teeth with the finger or a cotton tip applicator. Work on one quadrant at a time. Manipulate the dental tape between the middle fingers on each hand. Insert the tape obliquely into the contact area, using a back-and-forth motion and light pressure, and then wrap the tape around the tooth. Polish the proximal surfaces of each tooth with the tape, moving along adjacent teeth. Rinse and evacuate the patient's mouth. Remove any remaining residue with dental floss and subsequently rinsing. Use unwaxed floss if the dentist will follow with a fluoride application afterwards, because waxed floss coats the teeth and deters fluoride absorption.

## SELECTING AND MANIPULATING DENTAL FINISHING AND POLISHING AGENTS

**Finishing agents** include abrasives with a range of particles, beginning with coarse hard particles that are used to remove surface irregularities and to contour teeth and graduating to finer particles following a standard abrasive sequence with each abrasive rinsed completely from the teeth before use of a finer abrasive. Finishing may be used to smooth a surface after restoration. Agents include silicon carbide, aluminum oxide disks, flint, and iron oxide. Finishing abrasives are usually impregnated in plastic or paper discs for air-abrasion units. Finishing is usually combined with polishing to ensure that the surface is smooth, making the surface easier to clean and more resistant to corrosion. Fine **polishing agents** (abrasives 1-2 Mohs units harder than surface) may be used in discs or mixed with glycerine or water to make slurry. Polishing abrasives include calcite, Kieselguhr, pumice, rouge, silex, tin oxide, tripoli, zirconium silicate, and a number of prophylactic pastes. A slow speed should be used on the handpiece for polishing to minimize trauma.

## SELECTING AND MANIPULATING DENTAL CLEANING AGENTS

**Cleaning agents** are used primarily to remove staining, biofilms, and soft deposits (after hard deposits are removed). Cleaning agents include abrasives and chemicals. Cleaning may include coronal polishing, which helps to eliminate biofilms and staining, with a rubber polishing cup and a fine abrasive. Plaque and stain may be removed by air-powder polishing, which uses water and sodium bicarbonate under pressure. The flow rate is adjusted according to the degree of stain. Another method to remove plaque and stain is rubber-cup polishing (the most common method), with the abrasive agent placed in a small rubber cup on a handpiece. The cup rotates against the teeth. Premixed abrasives or reconstituted powder abrasives may be used, but if mixing, it's important for the mixture to be wet but not runny. Bristle brushes may be used to reach into pits/fissures on the tooth surface but may damage the gingiva. Cleaning abrasives include silex (heavy stains), super-fine silex (light stains), pumice (persistent stains), zirconium (cleaning/polishing), and chalk (whitening).

## ENAMEL SEALANTS

**Enamel sealants** are hard resins spread over occlusal surfaces of children's premolars or molars with no decay. Sealants bind to the pits and fissures on the occlusal surface to lock out possible decay for five to seven years. Both deciduous and permanent, including newly erupted teeth, can be sealed. Sealants are especially indicated for patients with many other occlusal caries or deep fissures. Fluoridate the teeth in conjunction with sealing. Enamel sealants are inappropriate for teeth that are:

- Decay-free for at least four years.
- Shallowly grooved, easy to clean, and decay-resistant.
- Well blended with pits and fissures.
- Already decayed.
- Restored.
- Resins enamel sealants are dilute concentrations of BIS-GMA dental composites or glass ionomers. They may be chemically cured two-paste systems or one-component light cured ones, and they may contain fluoride. Perform pre-etching and conditioning before application with phosphoric acid because the enamel binding is mechanical.

### PLACING ENAMEL SEALANTS ON CARIES-FREE TEETH

**Enamel sealing** is performed by the dental assistant with expanded functions.

1. Polish the occlusal surface to be sealed with flour of pumice or prophy paste without fluoride.
2. Use a rubber cup. Rinse and dry the area. Isolate it with a dental dam or cotton rolls.
3. Dab acid etchant/conditioner (phosphoric acid solution) over the occlusal surface into the pits and fissures to the upper two-thirds of the cusp, until the area looks chalky and white.
4. Rinse the tooth. Evacuate the mouth. Isolate tooth again with cotton rolls.
5. Prepare sealant according to the manufacturer's suggested procedure.
6. Place sealant into pits and fissures. Allow it to set (if self-curing) or light-cure it. Hold the curing light at the occlusal surface from 2 mm distance and expose it for up to one minute.
7. Test the hardness and smoothness of the sealant with an explorer.
8. Seal unsealed areas again, if necessary.
9. After setting, rinse or wipe the tooth surface.
10. Remove isolation materials. Check occlusion with articulating paper.
11. Gently finish. Apply fluoride.

## SUTURES

**Sutures** are surgical seams for closing wounds. Sutures support healing, and reduce contamination with pathogens and food debris. The dental assistant helps the dentist insert sutures. Some states permit assistants to remove sutures. Here are the types of dental sutures, from most common to least common:

- *Simple suture,* which is threaded through two skin areas and tied with a surgeon's knot.
- *Continuous simple suture,* which is a chain of sutures tied at either end with surgeon's knots, used for multiple extractions.
- *Sling suture* for interproximal areas, a threaded through the facial surface of the gum, enfolded around the lingual aspect of the tooth, put through the facial tissue on the other side of the tooth, wrapped back around the lingual side, and then the ends are tied.
- *Continuous sling variant* for a large opening, where the suture thread is wrapped onto the next tooth, instead of back around.
- *Mattress sutures* begin and end on the same aspect, e.g., the facial side, and the stitching is either horizontal or vertical.

## REMOVAL

Preparing for suture removal consists of the following:

- Remove sutures when healing is indicated, usually between 5 and 7 days after insertion.
- Set up a standard cart.
- Review the patient's chart.
- Debride the site using air and warm water spray, a cotton-tip applicator with water or dilute hydrogen peroxide, or moist cotton gauze.
- Inspect the suture site for location and number of sutures, the suture types and patterns, and healing of tissues in the region.
- For large areas with multiple extractions, healed areas look slightly red, with evidence of granulation tissue.
- If there was no periodontal dressing, there should be no infection.
- If periodontal dressing was performed, then a milky film should be in its place.
- For smaller areas where there was no periodontal dressing, the region should look fairly healed, with dark pink granulation tissue and no evidence of inflammation.
- Any wounds that are red, tender or bleeding are either infected, irritated or insufficiently healed.
- Confer with the dentist before suture removal.

### SIMPLE AND CONTINUOUS SIMPLE SUTURES

Use aseptic technique for all suture removal. The dental assistant may only perform suture removal if the procedure is covered in their state under dental assistants' expanded functions. Otherwise, the dentist removes sutures. Do not disrupt the healing process; if unsure, consult the dentist before attempting removal. Control hemorrhaging by applying pressure with a gauze sponge. Do not cut knots. Do not pull exposed sutures and knots through the patient's tissue. For **removal of simple or continuous simple sutures**, gently lift the suture away from the tissues using a cotton plier. Cut the thread below the knot with a suture scissors near the tissue. Catch the knot in the pliers and pull it out. Place the suture on a gauze sponge for counting at the end of the procedure. Cut and remove each suture in a series of continuous simple sutures individually.

### HORIZONTAL AND VERTICAL MATTRESS SUTURES

As with all other types of suture removal, **mattress suture removal** is performed by the dentist or delegated to the expanded-function dental assistant if the state in which they practice permits it. Horizontal mattress sutures are placed by horizontal stitching through one surface, followed by the same on the other aspect, and tying. Vertical mattress sutures have vertical stitching on each surface. Nevertheless, suture removal is similar for both. Lift the knot with cotton pliers. Sever the suture below the knot near the tissue. Make another cut close to the tissue on the other surface. Remove the suture by holding the knot with the cotton pliers and pulling up. Place the spent suture on the gauze sponge for later counting.

### SLING AND CONTINUOUS SLING SUTURES

As with all other types of suture removal, **sling removal** is performed by the dentist or delegated to the expanded-function dental assistant if the state in which they practice permits it. Using aseptic techniques, the sling suture is severed in two places and loosened on both sides of the tooth with cotton pliers. The knot is pulled up and cut close to the tissue. The thread on the other side of the tooth is lifted with the pliers and cut. Each thread is taken out with the cotton pliers by drawing it toward the wrapped side. For example, a sling suture entered from the facial side and wrapped around the lingual side is pulled toward the latter during removal. Sutures are placed on a gauze sponge for counting.

## INTERMEDIATE RESTORATIVE MATERIAL REQUIRED FOR TEMPORARY RESTORATIONS

Intermediate restorative material required for **temporary restorations** includes:

- *Zinc oxide eugenol-based materials:* This allows small amounts of eugenol to spread through the dentin to the pulp of the tooth. This may help with healing of the pulp by delivering some anesthetic and anti-inflammatory effects. Its sedative effects also help the pulp to relax after a procedure, which further aides in healing. This is only used in small quantities because large quantities of eugenol can have damaging effects on the tissue.
- *Calcium sulfate-based materials:* Used as a temporary filling material. Cavit is soft and sets once it is permeated with water. Cavidentin will set after being immersed in water for 24 hours. Both materials are equally effective.
- *Glass ionomer materials:* This bonds to dentin to form an affective seal. This also has antibacterial qualities due to its release of fluoride, low pH, and the presence of strontium and zinc in the cement.
- *Biodentine:* Used as a dentine substitute. This can stimulate tissue regeneration, which produces an adequate response from the pulp.

## IMPRESSION TRAYS

**Impression trays** document tooth areas. They are for diagnosis, making temporary dental crowns, or developing an indirect casting. Commercially-available stock or preformed trays are used for preliminary and final impressions and temporary needs. They are sold in various sizes and materials, including metal, Styrofoam, and tough plastic. Impression trays can cover the full arch, a half arch (quadrant tray), or just the front teeth (section tray). Some are perforated, so the impression material bonds with the tray. Customized trays specially made for an individual are made of lightweight resins, either light-cured, acrylic or thermoplastic. They are used for final impressions, making temporary restorations, or vital bleaching (external surface teeth whitening).

## PRELIMINARY IMPRESSIONS

An impression is a negative copy of teeth and adjacent structures. **Preliminary impressions** are diagnostic models for preparation of orthodontic and dental appliances, and provisional dental crowns. Impressions record tooth condition prior to and after treatment, especially for custom impressions. Preliminary impressions are created by the dentist or assistant (if legally allowed by the state) from alginate, a hydrocolloid comprised of potassium alginate and other compounds. Alginate is sold as a powder, to which the assistant adds an equal amount of water. The material first goes through a sol or solution phase that is liquid or semi-liquid. It proceeds to a gel or semisolid phase. Use 2 or 3 scoops of powder and equal measures of water for mandibular or maxillary impressions. Working time is 2 minutes for normal set and 1¼ minutes for fast set. Normal and fast sets have setting times of 4½ and 1 to 2 minutes, respectively.

## IDEAL ALGINATE IMPRESSION

**Alginate** has short working and setting times. To create an ideal alginate impression:

1. The dentist or assistant should be positioned so that insertion is quick and controlled.
2. The impression tray containing the alginate mixture is turned a bit initially, so the team can place a corner of it into the patient's mouth.
3. Retract the patient's cheek out of the way.
4. Slide the tray into the mouth.
5. Center it over the teeth.
6. Seat the back part of the tray before the front part, to prevent alginate flowing into the mouth and throat.
7. Push the tray into place very gently.
8. Pull the patient's lips out around the tray.
9. Hold securely in place until the alginate sets.

## FINAL IMPRESSIONS

**Final impressions** provide more precise definition of the teeth and surrounding structures of interest than preliminary impressions. Occasionally, alginate is used for final impressions, but more often elastomeric impression materials are chosen. Two compounds are mixed together to create the final elastomeric material: A base and a catalyst. The various choices are defined by their viscosity or capacity to flow. Light, regular and heavy body materials are increasing thick. Heavy body is the most commonly used. There are four types of final impression materials available: Polysulfide, polyether, condensation silicone, and addition silicone. In terms of stiffness and stability, the best choice is addition stone, followed by polyether.

**Making final impressions** is a two-person job. The assistant mixes. The dentist takes the impression. Mixing time is a minute or less for all final impression materials. Setting time averages 6 minutes for all, except polysulfide, which takes 10 to 20 minutes to set. If the base and catalyst come as two pastes, they are mixed either by swirling them together and smoothing them with a spatula, or by using an automix system. The automix system consists of extruder units with cartridges of the base and catalyst, which are mixed when a trigger is squeezed. Segregate the tooth for which the impression is taken by a retraction system. Rinse and dry. Insert a recently-mixed light-body impression material is into the sulcus, around the tooth, and into adjacent areas. Mix the heavy-body material and place it into the impression tray. Load it in place over the light-body material. After setting, remove the impression. Examine and disinfect it. Placed in into a labeled precaution bag for transport to the laboratory.

## GINGIVAL RETRACTION

**Gingival retraction** uses a cord to briefly push the gingival tissue away from a tooth and broaden the sulcus. Gingival retraction cords isolate a tooth for the final impression. Dry the tooth. Separate the quadrant with cotton rolls. Loop the retraction cord and slide it over the tooth. Push it into the sulcus in a clockwise motion with a cord-packing device. The end of the cord should end up on the facial side, where it remains sticking out; it may be placed into the sulcus. After several minutes, remove the retraction cord counterclockwise with cotton pliers. Dry the area and apply new cotton rolls. Procure the impression quickly. Sometimes, chemical retraction is used in conjunction with these procedures by initial use of a topical hemostatic solution, aluminum salt astringents, or epinephrine (an astringent and vasoconstrictor). Retraction can also be performed with a surgical knife or electric cauterizer.

## OCCLUSAL REGISTRATIONS

**Occlusal or bite registrations** are impressions that document the centric relationship between a patient's maxillary and mandibular arches. The centric relationship is the position of optimally stable connection between occlusal surfaces of the two arches when the mouth is closed. Bite registrations are made of wax or paste, both of which do not flow easily. If wax is used, heat it for softening. Place wax directly onto the occlusal surfaces. The patient bites down lightly into the wax until it cools. Remove the registration and store it Pastes set quickly, are odorless and tasteless, and conform easily to biting. Pastes have two cartridges or parts that are mixed. Spread right over the teeth or put in a gauze tray, and then the patient bites down for the impression.

## BITE REGISTRATIONS

**Bite registrations** are performed by the dental assistant under supervision, or by the dentist, aided by the assistant. Use either bite registration wax or polysiloxane. Sit the patient upright. Teach the patient how to bite in occlusion before the registration. If bite registration wax is used, determine the correct length, warm and soften it with water or a torch, and then place it on the mandibular occlusal edges. If polysiloxane is used, force the material through an extruder gun with disposable tip, right onto the occlusal surfaces. The assistant watches to ensure the patient bites with proper occlusion, as previously directed. The patient holds the occlusion for a minute or two, while the wax cools, or until the polysiloxane hardens. Remove the bite material. Disinfect and label the impression. Store it for later use.

## ARMAMENTARIUM REQUIRED FOR ORAL SURGERY

Armamentarium required for **oral surgery** includes:

- *Chlorhexidine gluconate:* Used as a one-minute pre-rinse to disinfect.
- *Surgery setup pack:* Necessary PPE, drapes, and covers.
- *Paper products:* Gauze, cotton rolls, cotton-tipped applicators.
- *Suction tips:* Sterilized tips for saliva ejector and suction.
- *Blood pressure cuff:* To monitor blood pressure during the procedure.
- *Basic setup:* 2 dental mirrors, 2 cotton pliers, a periodontal probe, a hemostat, suction holder, surgical scissors, retractors, and scalpels.
- *Local anesthetic:* Medications and syringes should be available.
- *Retractors:* Retracts soft tissues (cheek and tongue) to better visualize the oral cavity.
- *Bite block:* Holds the mouth open wide comfortably.
- *Periosteal elevators:* Used to release the soft tissue surrounding the tooth.
- *Forceps:* There are several different styles, each used for grasping tissue.
- *Rongeur forceps:* Used to cut bone.
- *Chisel and mallet:* Used to remove bone.
- *Bone file:* Used for final smoothing.
- *Burr and hand piece:* Used in the final step of removing bone.
- *Curettes:* Used to remove small amounts of soft tissue.
- *Suturing materials:* Used for closing the surgical wound.

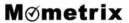

## CONTROL BLEEDING AFTER ORAL/DENTAL SURGERY

Methods to **control bleeding** after surgery include:

- *Compression:* A wet piece of gauze, or paper towel if the patient does not have gauze at home, can be folded and placed over the surgical site. The patient should then bite down to apply pressure for at least 45 minutes.
- *Elevation:* The patient should keep his head elevated above the level of his heart. Due to gravity, bleeding will increase when laying down or having the head dependent.
- *Black tea bags:* Wetting a black tea bag and biting down on it over the surgical site can decrease bleeding. Black tea contains tannic acid, which works as an anticoagulant and can decrease bleeding.
- *Rest:* Resting can decrease complications from oral surgery. Being overly active or engaging in strenuous activities can increase the risk for bleeding.
- *Be careful with eating and drinking:* Do not use a straw to drink liquids for several days following oral surgery because this can dislodge the blood clot and increase bleeding. Smoking, drinking carbonated or hot beverages, and eating rough or crunchy foods can also dislodge the clot and increase bleeding.

## POST-OPERATIVE COMPLICATIONS

The most common **post-operative complications** following oral surgery are dry socket and post-op infection.

- *Dry socket:* A dry socket develops when the blood clot after a tooth extraction is dislodged or dissolves. Risk factors include smoking, using a straw, poor oral hygiene, and birth control pills. The patient will have significant pain at the site or a sore throat. On exam, the GCA will see a dry socket without a blood clot and white bone. This is treated by cleaning the socket and placing a gauze strip impregnated with clove oil in the socket. If there is an increased risk for infection, the dentist may prescribe antibiotics.
- *Post-op infection:* Extensive oral surgery, poor oral hygiene, smoking, and diabetes are risk factors for post-op infection. There will be pain at the operative site and a bad taste in the mouth. On exam, the GCA will see redness and swelling at the surgical site, and there may be purulent drainage present. This often produces a bad odor. The dentist may prescribe antibiotics, or if severe, the wound may be opened and irrigated.

# Pain Management for Dental Procedures

## TOPICAL AND LOCAL ANESTHETICS

All **anesthetics** block nerve impulses, thus dulling pain sensations. The dentist or nurse spreads topical anesthetic directly over oral mucosa before injecting a local anesthetic. **Topical preparations** are usually ointments applied with a cotton swab, but they can be sprays, liquids, and patches. **Local anesthetics** are chemical amides and esters, and are injected in the proximity of the nerve associated with the tooth being treated. Local anesthetic agents have a particular timeframe after injection for induction of full numbing and later loss of numbing (duration). Local anesthetics are classified in terms of their duration as short-acting, intermediate-acting, or long-acting. Most procedures require the intermediate-acting duration of 2 to 4 hours. Most intermediate-acting and long-acting local anesthetic agents also contain small concentrations of vasoconstrictors, such as epinephrine, which decrease blood flow and bleeding to the region. These preparations are contraindicated in patients with hypertension, cardiovascular disease, liver or kidney disease, hyperthyroidism, or pregnancy.

## ASSISTING WITH ADMINISTRATION

The assistant prepares local anesthetic. The dentist dries the injection site with a sterile gauze sponge and applies topical anesthetic with a cotton swab for one minute. The assistant transfers the syringe to the dentist, either beneath the patient's chin or behind the patient's head. Pass the syringe with the thumb ring toward the dentist, the bevel of the needle facing the alveolar bone, and the protective cap secure but loose enough to remove during the transfer. The dentist performs the injection. The assistant observes the patient for adverse reactions. The dentist replaces the needle guard by scooping or uses a mechanical recapping device. If the patient requires additional anesthesia, the assistant swaps in a new cartridge and transfers it, as above. Replace the recapped syringe on the tray. Rinse and evacuate the patient's mouth at the conclusion of the procedure. Remove the capped needle by unscrewing or cutting it off and discarding it in the sharps container. Remove the cartridge by retraction of the piston and deposit it in a medical waste container. Sterilize the syringe.

## TYPES OF INJECTIONS FOR LOCAL ANESTHESIA

**Local anesthesia methods** fall into 3 categories:

- *Local infiltration* — The dentist injects the agent into gingival tissues near the small terminal nerve branches, numbing the necessary tooth and/or gums. The anesthetic can also be injected using pressure right into the periodontal ligament.
- *Field block* — The dentist injects the agent at the larger terminal nerve limbs near the apex of the tooth. The advantages of field block technique are avoidance of messages to the central nervous system and swift onset of action.
- *Nerve block* — The dentist introduces the agent close to a main nerve trunk, which eliminates pain sensations to the brain, and over a relatively large local area.

## ANESTHETIC SYRINGE

An **anesthetic or aspirating syringe** consists of the barrel, the disposable needle cannula, and the anesthetic cartridge. Both reusable stainless steel and disposable plastic syringes are available. The operator braces the thumb in a ring at one end and the index and middle fingers on grips. The barrel of the syringe is a long shaft, open on one side for cartridge insertion, with an observation window on the opposite side. Inside the barrel is a plunger or piston rod attached to a barbed-tipped harpoon at its end. There is a threaded tip at the end of the syringe, to which the sterile disposable needle (cannula) is attached. The cannula has a short cartridge end attached to needle hub, which is either pushed or screwed onto the threaded tip of the syringe. The slanted tip (bevel) on the other end penetrates tissue. The segment between is the shank; the solution travels through its internal, hollow lumen. Anesthetic cartridges containing the agent are made of glass. They have a rubber stopper end to attach to the harpoon of the syringe and an aluminum cap end for needle insertion.

## PREPARATION

The dental assistant is responsible for **preparation of the anesthetic syringe** outside the viewing area of the patient. Take the sterile syringe out of its autoclave pouch. Hold the syringe in the left hand. Withdraw the piston rod by pulling back on the thumb ring. With the right hand, position the rubber stopper end of the cartridge into the barrel of the syringe. Connect he harpoon to the rubber stopper using medium pressure on the finger ring. Take off the cap of the syringe end of the disposable needle and screw or push it onto the threaded tip of the syringe. Remove the needle guard. Check for correct operation by forcing out a small amount of reagent, while holding the syringe upright.

## CARE AND HANDLING OF ASPIRATING SYRINGE

Sanitize the harpoon of a stainless-steel **reusable aspirating syringe** after each use and autoclave the entire syringe. From time to time, lubricate parts or the harpoon may require exchange. Discard plastic syringes in a biohazard container. Discard the cannula into a sharps container after normal use, if there is any evidence of a broken seal, or if tissue penetration occurs more than four times. Anesthetic cartridges come in sterilized, sealed blister packs and should be stored at room temperature in a dark area. Inspect the cartridge before use. Discard a cartridge that has expired or has large bubbles, rust, corrosion, or extruded stoppers. Dispose of a used cartridge in a tamper-proof container approved by the pharmacist. Be aware that addicts scavenge garbage for residual drugs.

## CODING OF ANESTHETIC CARTRIDGES

**Anesthetic cartridges** labeled with the American Dental Association's seal of acceptance have standardized color codes on a band near the rubber stopper. Sometimes, the aluminum cap is also colored similarly, although it may be silver. There is unambiguous, black lettering on the cartridge, identifying the agent and concentration. Some other cartridges have colored writing on the side. The ADA-approved color schemes are as follows:

- Articaine 4% with epinephrine 1:100,000 – gold.
- Bupivacaine with epinephrine – blue.
- Lidocaine 2% either plain or with epinephrine 1:50,000 or 1:100,000 - light blue, green, or red, respectively.
- Mepivacaine 3% or 2% with levonordefrin 1:20,000 - tan or brown, respectively.
- Prilocaine 4% without or with epinephrine 1:200,000 - black or yellow, respectively.

## MAXILLARY LOCAL ANESTHESIA INJECTION SITES

Local infiltration or field block techniques desensitize individual **maxillary teeth** when injected near the apex of specific anterior teeth. A nasopalatine nerve block, in which the lingual tissue next to the incisive papilla is injected, numbs the front of the hard palate between the canines. The greater palatine nerve block uses injection near the second molar and in front of the greater palatine foramen to block sensations to the entire hard palate and soft tissues posterior to the canine. A maxillary nerve block is an anesthetic injection into the mucobuccal fold near the second molar, which blocks one entire oral quadrant, and the skin on that side of the nose, cheek, upper lip and lower eyelid. The anterior superior alveolar, middle superior alveolar, and posterior superior alveolar nerve blocks involve injection into the fold at the first premolar, fold at the second premolar, and near the apex of the second molar respectively; each affects two or three close teeth and tissues.

## MANDIBULAR LOCAL ANESTHESIA INJECTION SITES

Local infiltration or field block techniques desensitize individual **mandibular teeth** by injecting near the apex of specific anterior teeth. Nerve blocks numb larger areas. Introduction of anesthetic into the mucobuccal fold in front of the mental foramen is an incisive nerve block, affecting teeth from the central incisors back to the premolars and the cheeks. Inferior alveolar nerve block or mandibular block dulls an entire quadrant, including teeth, mucous membranes, the front portion of the tongue, mouth floor, and soft tissues. It involves injection into the mandibular ramus, behind the retromolar pad. Lingual nerve block means the anesthetic is introduced lingually to the mandibular ramus and next to the maxillary tuberosity, affecting the mandibular teeth, the side of the tongue, and lingual tissues on one side. Buccal nerve block means the agent is injected into the mucous membrane behind the last available molar just to numb buccal tissue. Mental nerve block involves an injection between the apices of the premolars, to target the premolars, canines, and close facial tissues.

## ALTERNATIVE METHODS OF ADMINISTERING LOCAL ANESTHETICS

One relatively painless and fast method is **intraosseous anesthesia**, in which the cortical plate of bone is first perforated using a solid needle connected to a slow handpiece. The anesthetic agent is then injected into the hole, using an 8 mm, 27-gauge needle.

**Periodontal ligament injection** entails insertion into the gingival sulcus. A special injection syringe is used; it is gun-like and the syringe is attached externally.

Another technique is **intrapulpal injection** right into the pulp chamber or root canal, using a 25-gauge or 27-gauge needle.

There are **computer-operated delivery systems** available for administration of local anesthesia, which offer the ability to control parameters, such as rate of delivery and pressure.

There are also systems that deliver **electronic impulses**, instead of chemical preparations, in cases where chemicals are contraindicated.

## NITROUS OXIDE SEDATION

Analgesics are agents that relieve pain without loss of consciousness. **Nitrous oxide ($N_2O$)** is an analgesic dispensed simultaneously with oxygen ($O_2$) gas through a small nosepiece, connected via tubing to a tank. The inhaled gases migrate through the nasopharynx, the respiratory chambers, and eventually reach the alveoli in the lungs. The gasses are exchanged between the alveoli and the blood plasma and red cells. The circulatory system transports the gases by the blood to the brain, where the analgesic effect is initiated. Nitrous oxide and oxygen together have mild pharmacologic activity in the central nervous system. They create a state of calmness for the patient, called sedation. The setup generally includes an inside mask for inhalation of the gases, an outer mask attached to an external reservoir bag, and a vacuum to carry away exhaled and excess gas.

### DISPENSATION AND MONITORING

Depending on the state, these functions may be done by the dental assistant under supervision of the dentist, or as a cooperative effort. The assistant is responsible for rechecking equipment, gas levels in the tanks, and preparing the patient. The dentist explains the procedure and hazards involved with the patient. Ask the patient to sign an informed consent form. Tilt the patient back in

114

the chair. Attach a sterile nitrous mask to the tubing. Connect it to the tanks. Place the mask over the patient's nose. Tell the patient to breathe slowly through his or her nose. When indicated by the dentist, administer oxygen alone for one minute, at a rate of at least 5 liters per minute, to determine the normal tidal volume. Administer nitrous oxide in 500 ml to 1-liter increments per minute, with equivalent reduction of oxygen flow. Observe patient response to determine the optimal mixture that provides sedation, without impeding cognition. The dentist gives local anesthetic a few minutes after nitrous oxide administration is initiated.

## PROCEDURES FOR RECOVERY

Turn off the nitrous oxide under the dentist's direction. Allow the patient to receive only oxygen for about 5 minutes to stave off diffusion hypoxia, the inadequate supply of oxygen to bodily tissues. Remove the patient's mask. Tilt the chair upright to avoid postural hypotension or fainting. Do not dismiss the patient until he/she feels clear-headed (usually a few minutes). Chart the nitrous oxide administration, including baseline levels of both gases, and the patient's reactions. A good method of judging the psychomotor ability of the patient is to give a Trieger test prior to administration and after recovery. The Trieger test involves connecting a pattern of dots. The patient completes the test in the upright position. Disinfect the connecting tubing after use. Depending on office procedures, the masks may be discarded, or given to the patient for later reuse.

## SAFETY CONSIDERATIONS

The American Dental Association suggests that personnel in dental offices who administer nitrous oxide be monitored twice a year by dosimetry or infrared spectrophotometry. Nitrous oxide is associated with infertility problems.

**Use nitrous oxide for:**

- Apprehensive patients
- Patient with sensitive gag reflexes
- Heart patients, who benefit from supplemental oxygen and reduction of stress

**DO NOT administer nitrous oxide to:**

- Pregnant women in the first trimester
- Infertile individuals undergoing in-vitro fertilization procedures
- Neurology patients
- Drug abusers
- Psychiatric patients
- Immunocompromised patients in danger of bone marrow suppression
- Mouth breathers

## PAIN

The type and location of pain can help to determine the pain's underlying cause. The certified dental assistant should record the exact description of the pain and the degree of pain using the 1 to 10 scale and response to treatment and/or pain medication. Different **types of pain** include:

- *Acute pain*: The central part of the tooth, the pulp, contains nerve endings, and when the pulp becomes inflamed, because of a cavity or infection, the patient may experience severe pain. The pain may be localized to one tooth or to an area of the mouth.
- *Hot/Cold sensitivity (short-duration):* This may result from an exposed root or a small or loose cavity and may occur for a short period after recent dental work.

- *Sharp pain with pressure*: This may indicate tooth decay or a loose filling.
- *Persistent pain after contact with hot/cold foods*: This type of pain often indicates that the root is dying and a root canal is necessary.
- *Aching in sinus areas*: This may indicate a problem in an upper back tooth or in the sinuses.

## PAIN AND ANXIETY CONTROL DURING DENTAL PROCEDURES

Before, during and/or after dental procedures, the dentist administers some type of **pain and anxiety control** to the patient. The dental assistant preps the supplies. The dentist can alleviate pain and anxiety by psychological methods, such as hypnosis and biofeedback, by chemicals, or by physiologic agents. The dentist can prescribe five types of pain relief:

1. *Antianxiety drugs* that relieve apprehension (e.g., Valium).
2. *Local or topical anesthetic* that dulls pain (e.g., lidocaine).
3. *Inhalation sedation* that induces a state of calm drowsiness (e.g., nitrous oxide $N_2O$).
4. *Intravenous sedation* (e.g., Versed, a benzodiazepine).
5. *General anesthesia* by Jorgensen technique, which induces unconsciousness (e.g., pentobarbital sodium, a barbiturate, mixed with Demerol, an opioid, and scopolamine, an anticholinergic).

## DISMISSAL OF DENTAL PATIENT

After the operator has finished the dental procedure, the dental assistant is responsible for rinsing and evacuating the patient's mouth. The assistant pulls the dental light aside, positions the dental chair to upright, removes fragments on the patient's face, and takes off the bib. The assistant instructs the patient to stay seated for a minute, in case he/she is dizzy as a reaction to anesthetic. The assistant places the used bib, evacuator, air-water syringe tips, and saliva ejector on the tray. The assistant either takes off the treatment gloves and washes his or her hands, or uses overgloves to immediately record procedures performed on the chart or electronically. The assistant collects the chart and radiographs. The assistant provides the patient with postoperative instructions and returns his or her personal items. The assistant leads the patient to the receptionist, who deals with later appointments and payments.

# Dental Conditions/Emergencies

## DENTAL EMERGENCIES INVOLVING FRACTURED TEETH

Broken teeth are addressed according the amount and type of breakage, the degree of discomfort, and age. The dentist usually gives a child with a broken tooth pulp treatment and a temporary restoration, with a follow-up assessment several months later. **Tooth fractures** involving the enamel alone need their rough edges smoothed. If the fracture involves both enamel and dentin, then the exposed dentin is covered with glass ionomer, calcium hydroxide, and a bonding agent for composite restoration. If the break extends down into the pulp, then pulp capping or removal is indicated. If the crown is cracked with exposure of pulp, then a root canal supplemented by posts and casts in the crown for stabilization and protection are probably necessary.

## HARD TISSUE DAMAGE IN ORAL CAVITY

**Hard tissue** is calcified tissue, such as bone, teeth, enamel, dentin, and cementum. The causes of damage to this material is most often traumatic. This can include a broken tooth from chewing on a hard substance or from a traumatic blow to the mouth. Tooth decay and lead to breakdown of the enamel on the surface of the teeth. Beneath the enamel, is a substance called dentin which can be damaged when enamel is broken down. Cementum is a hard substance that covers the roots of a tooth and this can be damaged when there a tooth is broken off or the roots are disrupted.

The most common symptom associated with **hard tissue damage** in the oral cavity is pain. When a tooth breaks, the inner nerves can be exposed which produces significant pain. Damage to a tooth can be visible if the exposed surface is broken. Damages to the root of the tooth can cause significant pain and swelling and redness at the gum line.

## TREATMENT FOR TRAUMA TO HARD TISSUE OF ORAL CAVITY

**Trauma to the hard tissues of the oral cavity** is considered a dental emergency. If the trauma is to a primary tooth, rather than a permanent tooth, the tooth will not be splinted or re-inserted. If the trauma is to a permanent tooth, the following steps should be taken:

- *Loose or displaced teeth:* Splinting is usually performed to reposition the tooth into its proper alignment. If the tooth is completed removed from its socket due to the trauma, it should not be handled by the roots. The tooth should be placed in milk until the dentist can evaluate. Reinsertion of the tooth is most successful if no more than 60 minutes has passed since the injury occurred.
- *Broken teeth:* If a primary tooth is broken, the tooth will likely be extracted. If a permanent tooth is broken, any fragments should be kept in milk until the dentist can evaluate the patient. The fragments may be viable to reattach to the permanent tooth.

## SOFT TISSUE INJURIES IN ORAL-FACIAL AREA

**Soft issue injuries** to the oral-facial area can occur easily during dental procedures because the oral cavity is damp and slippery, the patient may shift, or equipment can be dislodged. Soft tissue injuries to the area can also be caused outside the office by any contact with a sharp or dull object, electrical burns, or sports injuries. A situation unique to children is **traumatic intrusion**, the forcing of freshly erupted teeth back into their sockets after a tumble. Traumatic intrusion is treated by either permitting the teeth to re-erupt, or by moving them and using a splint across adjacent teeth for support. If traumatic intrusion occurs to primary teeth, the extent of damage to emergent permanent teeth underneath cannot be fully ascertained until they erupt.

## ABSCESSED OR AVULSED TEETH

**Abscesses** are pus-filled, inflamed cavities from bacterial infection. Abscessed teeth are hot and painful due to pressure and edema. Untreated infection spreads into the surrounding tissues, producing a fistula (passageway) leading from the oral cavity, which alleviates some of the pressure. The danger is infection of the meninges around the brain. Treatment is root canal therapy, removal of necrotic pulp, opening the pulp chamber, antibiotic therapy.

If the patient is conscious, wrap an avulsed permanent tooth in wet gauze and insert it between the teeth and lip. If the patient is unconscious or incapable, put the loose tooth in milk. Take patient and tooth to the dental office at once. The dentist then reattaches the tooth in the socket, using adjacent teeth to shore it up. Primary avulsed teeth are not reattached because infection or ankylosis (fusion of bone and cementum) can result. Primary teeth displaced to the side or loosened are repositioned and secured with a temporary splint as soon as possible.

## ALVEOLITIS

Normally, a blood clot forms over the socket where a tooth has been extracted. The clot protects the nerve endings and discourages infection. **Alveolitis** is a dry socket, where there is no blood clot formation, or the clot is rinsed out of the socket. Nerve endings are exposed and the extraction area is susceptible to infection. The therapy for alveolitis is cleansing with saline and stuffing the socket with a gauze strip or sponge drenched in the antiseptic iodoform to relieve pain. Analgesics may be used for palliation, such as ibuprofen. Medicated dressings are usually replaced in a day or two. In a surgical setting after extraction, anesthesia may be administered prior to alveolitis treatment.

# Diagnostic/Laboratory Procedures and Dental Materials

## General Dental Materials

### EFFECTS OF THERMAL PROPERTIES OF DENTAL MATERIALS ON THEIR USE

The important **thermal properties** of a potential dental material are its thermal conductivity and its thermal expansion. Thermal conductivity refers to the facility to convey heat. Materials with lower thermal conductivity are preferred usually particularly if they are near the dental pulp. Thermal expansion refers to the rate of expansion and contraction when exposed to temperature variations. It is important to select a material that has thermal expansion rates similar to that of tooth structure. Thermal expansion can cause dimensional changes in the dental material, particularly during the setting process. This can result in a phenomenon called microleakage in which debris and saliva leak into the area between the tooth and restorative material. Later, tooth sensitivity or caries can result.

### ROLE OF ACIDITY IN SELECTION OF DENTAL MATERIALS

The parameter pH is a measurement of the relative **acidity**, neutrality or alkalinity of a solution or environment. It is quantified on a scale from 0 to 14. Low numbers indicate acidic environments. pH 7.0 is neutral. High numbers indicate alkalinity. Normally, the oral cavity is maintained at relative neutrality by saliva. However, sugary and acidic foods and bacteria cause ongoing fluctuations in pH. Select dental materials to withstand these fluctuations. Some dental materials themselves are acidic and potentially damaging to gum tissues or pulp. If used, acidic materials must be set up and inserted cautiously.

### PROPERTIES OF DENTAL MATERIALS

Some important properties of dental materials to consider before selection include:

- **Adhesion** - The ability of dissimilar materials to stick together, either chemically or physically.
- **Elasticity** - The capacity to undergo distortion and return to the original conformation, such as rubber bands within their elastic limit.
- **Flow** - Gradual continual shape change under force, such as compression-associated amalgam changes.
- **Hardness** - Relative ability to resist scratching or denting.
- **Solubility** - Capacity to dissolve in fluid; extremely soluble materials are undesirable if in contact with saliva.
- **Viscosity** - Thickness or facility of a liquid to flow.
- **Wettability** - The capacity of a liquid (the dental material) to flow over and sink into another (the tooth).
- **Corrosiveness** - The ability to react with food or saliva causing pitting, coarseness or tarnishing, with metal-containing materials.
- **Galvanism** - Electric shock caused by reaction between dissimilar metals and carried by saliva.

## RETENTION

**Retention** is the act of keeping or holding something in place. In dentistry, retention is achieved by either mechanical or chemical means. Dental materials are held in place by mechanical retention by slanting the cavity walls inward, abrading the tooth surface with an etchant, or by furrowing the cavity walls. Chemical retention is achieved by some sort of chemical reaction between the dental material and the tooth surface. It is often used for insertion of gold inlays or crowns, which must be indirectly retained through use of cements or bonding agents.

120

Copyright © Mometrix Media. You have been licensed one copy of this document for personal use only. Any other reproduction or redistribution is strictly prohibited. All rights reserved. This content is provided for test preparation purposes only and does not imply an endorsement by Mometrix of any particular political, scientific, or religious point of view.

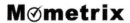

# Impression Materials and Procedures

## ALGINATE IMPRESSIONS

### MATERIAL

**Alginate** is a general term for **irreversible hydrocolloid impression materials.** These materials make impressions for diagnostic casts and study models. Their main application in orthodontic work is as negative models for preparation of casts that can be used to formulate orthodontic appliances. Hydrocolloid impressions are also taken to make opposite models for prosthetics, temporary restorations, bleach trays, custom trays, and mouth guards. The main ingredient is marine-derived potassium alginate. It is soluble in water, forming a thick liquid or sol. When calcium sulfate is added, solidification (a gel) occurs. Hydrocolloid impression materials also contain trisodium phosphate, which slows down setting time, fillers like diatomaceous earth or zinc oxide for strength, and potassium titanium fluoride.

### ADVANTAGES AND DISADVANTAGES

Alginate is extensively used because it is easy, cheap, and comfortable to use, it sets quickly, and little equipment is needed. Its elastic properties make it ideal for making impressions where there are recessed areas, and both tissue and teeth imprints can be taken. The major disadvantage is the possibility of some inaccuracy in the impression, due to changes in water content. Heat, dryness, or contact with air can result in syneresis or shrinkage of the material. Water gain can result in imbibition or an enlargement of the measurements of the impression. Tissue areas being imprinted may be distorted because of the thickness of the material. Other impression materials, such as elastomer, are more accurate.

### BOWLS, SPATULAS, AND TRAYS

Dispensing units using premixed units require only dispensing tips. The mixture is distributed directly into the tray. When mixing of the powder and water, use **flexible rubber bowls** and **throwaway spatulas** (generally two-sided for mixing of alginate or plaster). The bowl is sterilized or sanitized afterwards. There are also disposable spatulas and bowls with markings for water measurement. There are **metal impression trays** that must be sterilized after use and disposable plastic trays. Most have perforations to allow material through and keep it in place. There are also **unperforated rim lock trays** with rims to hold the impression material in place. Trays come in various sizes and should be selected so they fit the person's mouth, with room for 2 mm of the hydrocolloid. They should also reach several millimeters posterior to the molar area; if they do not, they can be extended using wax strips (beading).

### PREPARATION

If legally allowed by the state, the dental assistant can take **an alginate impression.** The patient should be sitting up, with mouth is rinsed and evacuated. Test the impression trays for size. If the selected tray does not extend beyond the molars, add wax beading to the borders. Prepare the mandibular model first. Add two measurements of room temperature water to one flexible mixing bowl, followed by two scoops of water in another bowl. Fluff the powder needs beforehand. Add the powder to the water and mix with the spatula, first by stirring, and then by applying pressure with the smooth side of the spatula on the side of the basin. Mixing time should be about 30 to 45 seconds for fast set, or 60 seconds for regular set preparations. A creamy, uniform consistency is desired. Put the preparation in the impression tray, starting from the lingual sides. The flat edge (and sometimes a moist, gloved hand) consolidates the material. Maxillary impressions, which have a greater tendency to cause choking, are prepared similarly later, except that 3 measurements of water and 3 scoops of powder are used.

## ACCURATE IMPRESSION

**Accurate alginate impressions** are centered over the central incisors, include all essential areas, and illustrate well-defined anatomic detail of both teeth and tissues. The teeth should not pierce through to the tray, caused by pushing the tray up or down too far. The imprint should not have tears, bubbles or empty spaces. It should encompass the vestibule regions and have a good peripheral or marginal roll. Certain features should be evident. For the mandibular impression, these are retromolar area, the lingual frenum and the mylohyoid ridge region. For the maxillary impression, these are the tuberosities and the palate regions.

## REMOVAL AND DISINFECTION OF ALGINATE IMPRESSIONS

Begin **removal of the alginate impressions** by using the fingers of one hand to break the seal between the tissues of the lips and the cheek and the tray. shield the opposite arch with the opposite hand. Abruptly remove the tray with a snapping motion, pulling up for the maxillary impression and down for the mandibular. Turn the tray a bit sideways for removal. Evacuate surplus alginate from the mouth. Tissue off surplus alginate from the face. Ask the patient to rinse and spit. Examine the impression for accuracy. Rinse it with tap water and spray it with an approved surface disinfectant, such as an iodophor. Alginate impressions that are not poured into casts immediately (within 20 minutes) should be enclosed in a labeled, covered container until use. If the impression is wrapped first in a moist towel, it leads to water intake and distortion over time.

# IRREVERSIBLE HYDROCOLLOID IMPRESSION MATERIALS

## SETTING TIMES

The period between which the water is added to the powder and the total setting of the mixture is the **gelatin time**. This includes approximately one minute of working time for Type II regular-set alginate and less for fast-set Type I. **Setting time** occurs after that, in approximately 1 to 2 minutes for Type I or 2 to 4½ minutes for Type II, if the impression is taken at normal room temperature, about 70 °F. Both working and setting times are shortened at higher temperatures and lengthened at lower temperatures, for example, with use of cool water. In general, Type I is useful for children or people who tend to gag, whereas the slower setting Type II is convenient for more difficult insertions or in situations where there is only one operator.

## STORAGE AND PREPARATION

**Irreversible hydrocolloid impression** materials or alginate may come packaged in:

- Hermetic plastic containers, with foil or plastic bags inside, containing the powder and measuring tools for water.
- Mixtures in sealed bags.
- Mixtures used with a dispensing unit.

Store irreversible hydrocolloid impression materials in areas where they will not be exposed to moisture or excessive heat. Shelf life is about one year. The method of mixing the powder and water is specified by the manufacturer. In general, the ratio between the two is 1:1, but two scoops of powder and two portions of water are used for mandibular impressions, while three of each is required for maxillary impressions. If too little water is added, the mixture will be too thick, and vice versa.

## REVERSIBLE HYDROCOLLOID IMPRESSION MATERIAL

### COMPOSITION AND USES

**Reversible hydrocolloid impression** material, also known as **agar-agar,** is similar in makeup to alginate. The difference is that hydrocolloid setting is achieved through a chemical reaction. The material is transformed from a gel to sol state by boiling for 10 minutes in a hydrocolloid conditioner unit. It is maintained in a liquid state in a 150 °F water bath until about 5 minutes before use, at which time it is moved to a 110 °F water bath. Further cooling to convert the material back to a gel occurs in the mouth, using hoses connected to the dental unit. Reversible hydrocolloid materials are quite accurate, making them useful for final impressions and other applications requiring detail. The disadvantages of hydrocolloid include the expense of additional equipment, longer preparation and setting (10 minutes), and distortion over time if exposed to environmental changes.

### PACKAGING AND EQUIPMENT

When **packaging reversible hydrocolloid impression materials**, use a three-compartment hydrocolloid conditioning unit. The separate sections all contain clean water maintained at different temperatures. Looking toward the unit, from the left the partitions are the boiling bath (150 °F, 66 °C), the storage bath (usually 110 °F, 45 °C), and the conditioning bath (water-cooled tray). The impression material is provided in collapsible plastic tubes or syringes, which are shuttled between the three compartments after the appropriate time. If tubes are used, they are positioned upside down, with tips tightly in place in each compartment. Syringes have special holding cases for the cartridge. Time must either be set digitally or watched by the dental assistant, particularly the boiling time (10 minutes) and conditioning bath (5 minutes). The tray must be cool enough for insertion to avoid burning the patient's mouth. Otherwise, taking the hydrocolloid impression is similar to use of alginate, except that the setting time is longer, about 10 minutes.

## ELASTOMERIC IMPRESSION MATERIALS

**Elastomeric impression materials** are more flexible than other types. This means they are less prone to tearing and distortion upon removal. They are also relatively impervious to temperature changes. There are three general types of elastomeric impression materials: Polysulfide, silicone, and polyether. Each type is prepared by mixing a catalyst or accelerator and a base material, engendering a process called polymerization. During the polymerization process, the material converts from a paste into a rubber-like, elastic mass. Elastomeric impression materials are mixed using either a mixing pad and spatula, or an extruder gun, to which cartridges of base and catalyst and a mixing tip are attached externally.

### POLYSULFIDE IMPRESSIONS

**Polysulfide impressions** are taken by the dentist, supported by one or two assistants. The patient is sitting up. Rinse and evacuate the patient's mouth. Two different mixtures are prepared by separate individuals: One mixture for loading onto a syringe, and another for loading onto the impression tray. Parallel, non-touching lines of base and accelerator pastes are dispensed onto two paper pads. Each is mixed using a spatula, with the mixing of the syringe preparation initiated about a minute before that for the tray. Place the syringe preparation into an impression syringe that has an attached tip. Remove the cylinder by forcing it into the barrel, using the working end. Insert the plunger. Transfer the syringe to the dentist, who applies the material to the prepared tooth. Load the tray mixture into the impression tray with a spatula, smooth it out, and pass it to the dentist for insertion. Hold the tray in place for setting, a minimum of 6 minutes. Clean the spatula by pulling the material off, followed by sterilization. Discard the paper sheet and disposables.

## SILICONE IMPRESSIONS

To being the **two-step silicone impression**, the dental assistant supports the dentist. The patient sits erect. Don vinyl gloves. Silicone impression materials come as two color-coded putties and scoops (base and catalyst), or a putty base and catalyst in liquid dropper form. Blend equal amounts and mold them into a homogenous patty. Load the patty into a stock tray with adhesive, within 30 seconds. Forge a dent where the affected teeth are to be placed. Place a plastic spacer sheet over the tray and place it in the patient's mouth. Remove the tray and spacer after about 3 minutes and allow the preliminary impression to set. Position a retraction cord over the desired tooth, in preparation for the final impression. Use an extruder gun because it mixes and dispenses a lighter body silicone preparation. Force some of the material through a mixing tip into the preliminary impression tray. Use an intraoral delivery tip to inject some material around the prepared tooth, after retraction cord removal. The dentist places and holds the tray in place a minimum of 3 minutes until set. Remove the impression, rinse, gently dry, and disinfect it.

## POLYETHER IMPRESSIONS

When taking a **polyether impression**, first spread the two pastes, containing the base and catalyst, in parallel lines onto a paper pad. Quickly mix them for 30 seconds or less, using a spatula. Put the paste into the impression tray and hand it to the dentist for the preliminary impression. The dentist positions the tray and holds it about 3 minutes in the patient's mouth before removal. About 2 minutes into this process, the tray is moved around. For the final impression, the base, catalyst, and sometimes a consistency modifier (for thinning) are mixed and forced into the open end of an injection syringe. This material is put into the preliminary impression, and the tray is reintroduced into the patient's mouth. Hold it in the mouth about 4 minutes. Remove it abruptly with a snapping motion. Rinse, dry, and disinfect the impression for 10 minutes with 2% glutaraldehyde. Sometimes, only final polyether impressions are made.

## PROS AND CONS OF EACH TYPE

The **pros and cons of elastomeric impression materials** are:

- *Polysulfide* - It comes as a two-paste system, with a base of thiokol polysulfide rubber and filler and a catalyst of lead peroxide. Material is stable after setting, very precise, and has a long shelf life. However, it has a sulfurous odor, stains, and long setting time (at least 10 minutes).
- *Silicone* - It comes as two color-coded putties, a base of polysiloxane or polyvinyl siloxanes, and a catalyst. The putties are mixed and dispensed using an extruder gun. Silicone impression materials are highly accurate, stable, odorless, tasteless, and do not shrink or change measurements. They are relatively expensive.
- *Polyether* - It comes as a color-coded two paste system. The pastes (base and catalyst) are spread in parallel on a paper pad and mixed with a spatula. Polyether systems are quite accurate and stable.

# Restorative Dental Materials and Procedures

## IN-OFFICE BLEACHING AND HOME BLEACHING

Teeth can be bleached to remove both extrinsic stains from habits like coffee-drinking, and intrinsic stains from root canals, tetracycline use, damage, or fluorosis. Use sodium perborate, hydrogen peroxide, or carbamide peroxide. **In-office bleaching of vital teeth** is performed by the dentist with assistance. Smear protective gel on adjacent tissues. Isolate the area with a dental dam and a ligature of waxed floss surrounding each tooth. Polish teeth crowns with pumice or prophy gel. Mix bleaching materials according to the manufacturer's directions until thick. Apply directly onto the facial and lingual facades of the teeth or in a tray. Some materials require use of heat or light, or reapplication of fresh gel every 10 minutes. After bleaching, rinse. Remove the dam and ligatures. Polish teeth with a resin polishing cup or prophy paste containing fluoride. Home bleaching involves taking an alginate impression, from which a cast and custom trays are made. The patient uses the trays at home with a bleaching kit, as directed.

## NON-VITAL BLEACHING OF TEETH

**Non-vital bleaching** means lightening endodontically treated (usually root canal) or non-vital teeth. The dentist bleaches teeth with assistance. Apply protective gel to soft tissues. Place a dental dam and a ligature of waxed dental floss around the indicated tooth or teeth. The dentist removes the crown restoration and debris and may scrub the open crown. The dentist applies a 2 to 3 mm layer of base cement, light-cured resin ionomer, or bonded composite to the top of the root canal to ensure bleach does not enter the root. There are two options for the actual non-vital bleaching:

- *Gel bleaching* in the office, which entails filling the chamber with bleaching gel for 30 minutes, with bleach changes every 10 minutes (and possibly heat application), followed by cotton roll isolation and placement of a temporary crown. Requires 3 appointments spaced 3 to 7 days apart.
- *Walking bleaching*, this is placement of a viscous paste of hydrogen peroxide and/or sodium perborate into the crown and covering it with temporary cement. Requires 3 appointments, space 2 to 5 days apart.

Finally, remove the temporary filling and install the permanent filling. Veneers may be indicated.

## PREPARING, DELIVERING, MIXING, AND STORING OF DENTAL MATERIALS

The preparing, delivering, mixing, and storing of the following dental materials:

- **Bleaching Agents** - Carbamide peroxide and/or hydrogen peroxide in various concentrations (usually 15-38% for office and 3 to 15% for home). Typical preparations are in premixed gel form in tubes or prefilled applicators and must be stored at room temperature.
- **Bonding Agents** - Resins used to adhere dental composite materials. Many different bonding agents (with or without etchants) are available. Some are universal but others are specific to the type of material to which it will bond. Some are light-cured, and some vary in strength of bonding depending on the substrate. Some require more than one layer, some have strong odor, and some require longer curing time. Dry storage at room temperature.
- **Pit/Fissure Sealants** - Plastic coating to fill in grooves, pits, and fissures in chewing surfaces of back teeth to decrease the risk of bacterial buildup. A variety of sealants include resin-modified glass ionomer cements, glass ionomer cements, fluoride-releasing composites, and adhesives. They may last for up to 10 years. Dry storage.

## BONDING AGENTS

**Bonding agents** are materials that adhere restoration materials to either dentin or enamel. They are also referred to as adhesives or bonding resins. The main constituents of bonding agents are low-viscosity resins and sometimes fillers, enhancers, or fluoride. Most preparations are light-cured or dual-cured. In order for bonding to occur, surface alteration or scoring needs is performed before the bonding agent can penetrate the surface and form a mechanical bond. For enamel bonding, the first step is acid etching using phosphoric acid. Bonding to the more sensitive, organic and water-filled dentin is achieved by initially slashing the dentin with a burr, and then using an etchant to eliminate the resulting smear layer.

### PLACEMENT

**Bonding systems** consist of the acid etchant, primer or conditioner, and the adhesive or bonding agent. The dental assistant is responsible for preparation and transfer of materials and maintenance of a dry and clean area. If the procedure is in close contact with the pulp, the first step is placement of lining cement, such as calcium hydroxide. The etchant is then applied to the enamel and then the dentin. Manufacturer's instructions indicate the correct application time. The tooth is rinsed. A brush or disposable applicator is used to apply a primer, which moistens the dentin, and seeps into the tubules. The bonding agent is then placed and solidified, using a curing light. Disposable tips or brushes are thrown away.

## DENTAL CEMENTS

**Dental cements** are agents that bond other dental materials, like restorations to the teeth. Cements come in various forms that generally require mixing and preparation before use. The cements are hardened either by chemical self-curing or light curing with a special blue light. Cements are defined as temporary, intermediate, or permanent, depending on their expected duration. There are also thin liners that are used to seal and protect the pulp or wall and floor of the cavity. Bases are relatively strong dental cements that are thickly spread in a layer between the tooth and restoration for pulp protection. Besides restorations, cements are also utilized as luting or bonding agents to apply orthodontic bands, bridges, or inlays to the teeth.

Most **dental cements** are permanent, including zinc phosphate, reinforced zinc oxide eugenol, polycarboxylate, glass ionomer, resin cement, resin-reinforced glass ionomer, and compomers. The cements that are used for permanent cementation of orthodontic bands and brackets are zinc phosphate, polycarboxylate, glass ionomer and resin cement, all of which are bases and used to cement crowns, inlays, onlays and bridges. Glass ionomer is also utilized to seal root canals and for restorations. Reinforced zinc oxide eugenol is not used for orthodontic work. Resin cement is employed for cementation of enzootic posts, ceramic or composite inlays and onlays, and resin-bonded bridges. Compomers are resins altered with polyacid. Resin-reinforced glass ionomer is used for metallic or porcelain-fused metallic restorations. Zinc oxide eugenol is used only for temporary cementation of crowns, inlays, onlays and bridges, as a root canal sealant, or as a periodontal dressing after surgery. Varnish and calcium hydroxide are examples of liners.

## ZINC PHOSPHATE CEMENTS

**Zinc phosphate cement** preparations are composed of two parts that are mixed together. The first is a powder made of zinc oxide, and a small quantity of magnesium oxide, and tints of white, yellow or gray. The second part is a buffered phosphoric acid solution. When the two are combined, a heat-liberating or exothermic reaction occurs, which must be dampened during preparation by using a cooled glass slab and spatula. The mixture hardens within about 5 minutes and is very strong. The mechanism of bonding is mechanical interlocking. The desired consistency depends on the use; it should be creamy in texture for luting and similar to thick putty for use as a base.

## MIXING ZINC PHOSPHATE CEMENTS

The dental or orthodontic assistant mixes the **zinc phosphate cement** on a clean, cooled glass slab. The powder portion is spread, flattened, and divided with a stainless-steel cement spatula on one end of the slab. The liquid portion is dispensed with the dropper bottle unto the other end. The flat side of the spatula is used to integrate a portion of the powder into the liquid for about 15 seconds. The mixture is spread over a larger area of the slab and slowly more powder is mixed in with the spatula until the desired thickness is achieved. The mass is formed into a ball and transferred to the dentist on the slab under the person's chin. The assistant also transfers a plastic filling instrument to the dentist. The slab and spatula are wiped with moistened gauze, soaked in water or bicarbonate, and then sterilized or disinfected.

## ZINC OXIDE EUGENOL CEMENTS

**Zinc oxide eugenol (ZOE)** cement comes in two types. The traditional type I preparation consists of a powder containing zinc oxide, zinc acetate, resin, and an accelerator, which are mixed with the liquid eugenol. ZOE is used only for temporary cementation or for post-surgical periodontal dressing because of its soothing properties. The variant type II preparation is reinforced with alumina and other resins and alumina in the powder and ethoxybenzoic acid in the eugenol and it is useful for up to a year as an Intermediate Restorative Material (IRM). Zinc oxide eugenol is very soluble and of neutral pH. When reinforced, ZOE is also strong. ZOE is incompatible with acrylic or composite restorations. Mixing is done on either a paper pad or glass slab, using a stainless-steel cement spatula. Eugenol disintegrates rubber, so it should not meet the bulb. ZOE preparations are not used for orthodontic procedures.

## MIXING THE POWDER/LIQUID FORM

For **mixing powder/liquid zinc oxide eugenol (ZOE)** the dental assistant dispenses the powder onto the mixing pad (paper or glass), followed by the liquid. The two should be placed near but not on top of each other. Mix the two with the cement spatula, using the flat part of the instrument and uniform pressure. Consolidate the mixture into a mass to check for consistency, which should be creamy for luting applications, and similar to putty if needed as an insulating base or intermediate restorative material. Transfer the material to the dentist under the individual's chin, using a plastic filling instrument. Wipe off both the spatula and plastic filling instrument after use. If a paper pad was used, remove the top paper. If a glass slab was used, clean it with alcohol or orange solvent.

## MIXING THE TWO-PASTE SYSTEM

For **mixing the two-paste system of zinc oxide eugenol cement,** the dental assistant mixes and distributes pastes. If state law allows, the assistant can place pastes. If the law does not allow this extended responsibility, the assistant aids the dentist in placement of these preparations. Two-paste systems are used for temporary bonding. They consist of an accelerator and a base. Each paste is spread parallel to the other along a paper pad. A cement spatula is used to mix the two until they have a creamy texture, suitable for luting. This process is very fast (about 15 minutes), as is the setting time (5 minutes or less). The material is put in place with the plastic filling instrument. The cement spatula is wiped off with a gauze sponge.

## POLYCARBOXYLATE CEMENTS

**Polycarboxylate cements** are mainly used for permanent cementation of orthodontic bands and brackets. Polycarboxylate cements consist of two portions, which are mixed. The first is a powder, containing primarily zinc oxide, with smaller amounts of magnesium oxide and stannous fluoride. The second is a thick liquid made of polycyclic acid copolymer in water. Polycarboxylate cements adhere chemically to the teeth and mechanically to the restoration. They are relatively strong and non-irritating to the pulp. The chemical reaction does not release heat. These cements must be prepared and used quickly, as they have a mixing time of a minute or less and operational time of approximately three minutes, after which unutilized cement should be discarded when it appears dull or sinewy.

## PROCEDURES FOR MIXING

When **mixing polycarboxylate cements**, the dental assistant mixes cement. Place powder on one side of a paper pad or glass slab and drops of the liquid on the other. Manufacturer's directions should indicate the ratio of drops to scoops of powder. The relative amount of water is less if a base consistency is desired, or if the preparation is to be used for bonding. The powder is quickly incorporated into the liquid with some pressure for wetting. The mixture should have a glossy texture. For luting purposes, it should adhere to the spatula somewhat if raised an inch. It should be stickier for use as a base. The mixture should be applied within about 3 minutes, before it develops a dull and/or sinewy appearance. The spatula is wiped off with wet gauze, or bathed in 10% NaOH, if the cement has dried. Dispose of the paper pad.

## GLASS IONOMER CEMENTS

There are five types of **glass ionomer cements**:

- *Type I* is conventional, viscous, or condensable. It has fine grains and chemically binds to the tooth. Use it for orthodontic bonding and closing fissures and pits.
- *Type II* is conventional modified with resin by the addition of HEMA. It is coarser and is for restorations.
- *Type III* is dual-cured hybrid for luting.
- *Type IV* is tri-cured glass for opaque structures. It releases less fluoride than conventional glass ionomers.
- *Type V* is any metal reinforced admixture containing glass ionomers; it is used with silver or amalgam restorations for crown or core buildups.

Unless reinforced, these cements come as a silicate glass powder containing calcium, fluoride and aluminum, and an aqueous suspension of polycyclic acid. Glass ionomer cements are quite strong. They bond both chemically and mechanically to the teeth, discharge fluoride, and are relatively non-irritating. While the setting and working times are short, about 1 and 2 minutes respectively, these cements do not set completely for about a day. Resin-reinforced glass ionomer cements are stronger, less water-soluble, and more adherent.

## PROCEDURES FOR MIXING

When **mixing the glass ionomer cement**, the dental assistant first rinses and evacuates the patient's mouth. Dispense the powder and then the liquid portions onto a paper pad or cool glass stab. Immediately recap the liquid to avoid evaporation. Work quickly. Move a portion of the powder into the liquid with a flexible stainless-steel spatula. Mix and incorporate the remaining powder until the proper consistency is achieved. If the cement is for luting orthodontic work, the texture should be creamy and glossy. If it is a base, then the consistency should be stickier. Transfer the mixture to the dentist under the patient's chin along with the plastic filling instrument. Cleanup involves wiping off the instruments with a moistened gauze and disposal of the top paper. If glass ionomer capsules are used instead, the seal between the powder and liquid sides is broken in an activator and the tablets are mixed for about 10 seconds on an amalgamator. Place the capsule in a dispenser and transfer it to the dentist for application. Discard the remainder and disinfect the equipment.

128

## CALCIUM HYDROXIDE CEMENTS

**Calcium hydroxide cements** are placed in thin layers to protect the pulp by gently chafing the pulp enough to encourage secondary dentin formation. They are also used as liners under restorations. Calcium hydroxide cements are not very strong. Their formulations contain other chemicals, in addition to the calcium hydroxide, and may be either self-curing or light-curing. The most common system consists of two pastes, one of which is the base, and the other the catalyst for the reaction. With a two-paste system, equivalent small quantities of base and catalyst are dispensed onto a paper pad. The two are blended quickly (up to 15 seconds), using a small ball-ended instrument or explorer and a circular motion, until a consistent color is achieved. The assistant transfers the on the pad to the dentist under the patient's chin. The duration before setting can be from 2 to 7 minutes, depending on the preparation. The assistant wipes the instrument between applications and afterwards discards the paper pad.

## RESIN CEMENT

**Resin cements** are made up of bisphenol A-glycidyl methacrylate (BIS-GMA) or dimethacrylate resins, in combination with low-viscosity monomers, and sometimes fluoride. The cements do not bond directly to metal or ceramics. Instead, an etchant must first be applied to the tooth surface, or a silane coupling agent must be used to achieve mechanical or chemical bonding, respectively. Resin cements have a variety of applications. The curing method is related to the application. Self-curing or chemical-cured cements, which have an initiator and activator that are mixed, are used with metal restoration materials or endodontic posts. Orthodontic brackets and porcelain/resin restorations or veneers indicate use of light cured materials, which are supplied in syringes. There are also dual-cured materials that come in two parts, which are mixed, applied, and light-cured. There are polyacid-modified compomer cements with similar properties.

### DUAL-CURING TECHNIQUE FOR PLACEMENT OF ETCHANT AND RESIN CEMENT

When placing etchant and resin cement using a **dual-curing technique**, clean the tooth surface beforehand. Segregate the site with cotton rolls. The dental assistant prepares the etchant applicator and holds it on the tooth surface, per manufacturer's specifications, up to 30 seconds. The etchant may be transferred to and applied by the dentist. With the dual-curing method of resin cement placement, the tooth is then dried and the adhesive applied. The assistant quickly mixes resin components, initiator, and activator on a paper pad with a stainless-steel spatula to a uniform, creamy consistency. The assistant transfers the pad near to the patient, along with the plastic filling instrument. The placement is performed by the dentist. The assistant sets up the curing light. Actual curing or hardening may be done by the dentist or assistant, using the curing light and a protective shield or glasses when the light is on. Gauze sponges are used for cleanup and disposables are thrown out.

## ENDODONTIC MATERIALS AND ETCHANTS

### ENDODONTIC MATERIALS

**Irrigants** (sodium hypochlorite 1-10%, chlorhexidine gluconate, saline), **refrigerant spray** (for pulp testing), **lubricants**, **intra-canal medications** (paramonochlorophenol, polyantimicrobial paste), **fill material** (silver bulk fill, dental amalgam, medicated pastes, polyester resin), and **sealants.** Dry storage. Refrigerant spray must be stored in well-ventilated locked space as it may explode if overheated and may cause suffocation if inhaled.

### ETCHANTS

37% phosphoric acid used to etch a tooth before applying bonding. Many products are now self-etching and do not require separate etching but are rubbed on the tooth for 15 seconds and then air-dried. Some self-etching bonding agents come in two bottles with a drop or two placed on the tooth from each bottle or solutions mixed together prior to application. Dry storage.

## SURGICAL AND POST-EXTRACTION DRESSINGS, AND SEDATIVE DRESSINGS

**Surgical and post-extraction** dressings include:

- *Cellulose dressings* (Surgicel®, Benacel®, SureStop®) are absorbable cellulose hemostatic agents in sheets or plugs that are applied to the socket and create a gelatinous pseudo-clot. Cellulose dressings require dry storage and are packaged in individual sterile packets or blister packs.
- *Light-activated surgical dressing gel* (Barricade®) supplied in a disposable syringe for easy application. Dry storage.
- *Absorbable collagen* (OraTape, OraMem, OraCote): Packaged in plugs and sheets in sterile packages. Sheets can be cut to size and sutured into place and absorb over 10 to 14 days. Dry storage.

**Sedative dressing** is a mixture of clove oil and zinc oxide that is used as a temporary filling when restoration cannot be completed in one setting or when the decay is at or near the nerve to allow the tooth time to begin healing. Zinc oxide powder is mixed with the a few drops clove oil to make a very thick paste that is malleable but not sticky. Commercial products are also available. Ingredients are stored at room temperature.

## CAVITY VARNISH

**Cavity varnishes** close up dentin tubules before an amalgam restoration. They are applied in a thin layer to the dentin. All preparations contain some type of resin. Place universal varnishes under any restoration materials. Varnishes that include organic solvents are called copal varnishes, which are only appropriate under metal fillings. Varnishes are one of the weakest types of restorative materials, but they are impenetrable to oral fluids and are useful against microleakage or infiltration of cement acids into the dentin. The dental assistant prepares cavity varnishes. One's state may allow the dental assistant to apply varnish, or may stipulate the dentist does. The patient's mouth should be clean and dry. Apply two coats of varnish using two small cotton pellets and two cotton pliers. While holding it in the pliers, moisten the first pellet with the varnish. Recap the varnish to avoid evaporation. Dab away extra varnish with gauze. Coat the desired surface using the cotton pellet. After drying, repeat the procedure with the second pellet and pliers. Discard pellets. Wash the pliers with solvent.

## DENTAL BASES

**Dental bases** are intermediate restorative materials that are placed between the restoration and the dentine to protect the pulp. This is usually applied in a fairly thick layer to provide adequate protection. The dental base provides thermal insulation at the floor of the cavity and absorbs occlusal forces.

There are several different types of compounds used in creating dental bases:

- *Zinc oxide eugenol*: This may help with healing of the pulp by delivering some anesthetic and anti-inflammatory effects. Its sedative effects also help the pulp to relax after a procedure, which further aides in healing.
- *Zinc phosphate*: May be used to serve as a cement base for metallic restorations.
- *Glass ionomer*: Bonds to dentin to form an affective seal. This also has antibacterial qualities due to its release of fluoride, low pH, and the presence of strontium and zinc in the cement.

- *Polycarboxylate*: Primarily used for porcelain restorations, but can be used as a base for metallic restorations.
- *Flowable resin*: The dentin canals should be adequately sealed before using this to prevent irritation of the pulp.

## DENTAL LINERS

**Dental liners** are usually used over exposed dentine within the base of a cavity. While bases are generally applied in a thick layer, dental liners are usually applied in a thin layer. The liner effectively seals the dentine for protection, provides thermal insulation, and can help to stimulate the formation of irregular secondary dentine to aid in healing. These actions help to promote healing and prevent infection.

There are two different types of compounds used in creating dental liners:

- *Glass ionomer*: Usually used in a paste-liquid form, this forms a strong bond to dentin to form an affective seal, which can prevent micro-leakages. This also has antibacterial qualities due to its release of fluoride, low pH, and the presence of strontium and zinc in the cement.
- *Calcium hydroxide*: This has aides in producing an irregular secondary dentine to aid in healing and can prevent infection. Because of its poor strength properties, it cannot be applied in a thick enough layer to provide thermal for the pulp.

# Laboratory Materials and Procedures

## DENTAL WAXES

There are five categories of **dental waxes**:

- *Pattern wax* is composed of two hard waxes, inlay and baseplate. Inlay wax comes in dark sticks that are melted and placed on a die to create a pattern for a restoration, or heated to vaporization with the lost wax technique. Baseplate wax comes in sheets that are heated for use as denture bases.
- *Temporary processing waxes* include soft boxing wax, sticky wax, and utility wax. Soft boxing wax encloses impressions to keep gypsum in place. Sticky wax adheres to many types of surfaces when melted for temporary repair jobs. Utility wax has adhesive and malleable properties at room temperature, making it ideal for relieving patient discomfort. For example, place it over orthodontic brackets to making wearing more comfortable.
- *Impression or bite registration waxes* incorporate copper or aluminum particles.
- Hard blocks of study wax that can be whittled.
- *Undercut wax*, which is placed in undercuts before making impressions.

## GYPSUM MATERIALS

**Gypsum materials** are used to make impressions for dental models. All gypsum products are made from mined hard rock, heated to remove water in a process known as calcinations, which changes the ratio of calcium sulfate to water from 1:2 to 2:1 (from calcium sulfate dihydrate to hemihydrates). The resultant material is pulverized and colored; the particle size and color are indicative of the type of gypsum product. Finely ground gypsum materials are denser, stronger, and require less water for wetting and setting. When water is added to the particles, they convert back to the dihydrate form, discharging heat in an exothermic reaction. Setting is virtually complete when the model is cool to the touch, although complete setting may take a day. The setting time is conversely related to the water temperature. The water-to-powder ratio is crucial, as it determines strength and fluidity, and cannot be changed once setting has begun.

There are five types of **gypsum dental products**. Proceeding from Type I to Type V, the particles are finer, denser, stronger, and require less water for optimal setting.

| Type | Main Use | water per 100 g of powder |
|------|----------|---------------------------|
| Type I | Impression plaster for impressions | 60 mL |
| Type II | Model or laboratory plaster for casts/models | 50 mL |
| Type III | Laboratory stone | 30 mL |
| Type IV | Die stone for strong or dyed models | 24 mL |
| Type V | High-strength, high-expansion die stone | 18 to 22 mL |

Orthodontic stone is a combination of Type II laboratory plaster and Type III laboratory stone. Plaster is calcinated by an open kettle technique, making the particles very irregular and permeable. Die stone is processed by autoclaving with calcium chloride, making it denser and more uniform. Stone is alpha-hemihydrate. Plaster is beta-hemihydrate.

## DIAGNOSTIC CASTS

A **diagnostic cast** is a positive mock-up of the teeth and surrounding structures created by filling in the impression with model plaster or dental stone. Model plaster is the weaker material and is more easily trimmed. It is related to plaster of Paris. Dental stone is more robust and is the material of choice for retainers and custom trays. Both model plaster and dental stone contain gypsum, but a higher proportion of water is added to set model plaster than dental stone, or its stronger relative, high-strength stone. Setting time is affected by the type of gypsum, the water-powder ratio, length and speed of mixing, water temperature, and ambient humidity. Reduce setting time with a lower water-powder ratio, long or intense mixing, water temperature above room temperature, or on a humid day. Use the double-pour, box-and-pour, or inverted-pour methods. Trim and finish using a model trimmer. The end-product has two portions: An anatomic part showing the teeth, mucosa and muscle attachments (2/3), and an art portion or base (1/3).

## PROSTHODONTICS

**Prosthodontics** are artificial parts (*prostheses*) created in the dental laboratory to replace missing teeth or tissues. They can be fixed or removable. Fixed prostheses are designed to integrate into the natural dentition and are maintained through regular brushing and flossing. The purposes they serve include restoration of chewing ability, prevention of teeth movement by providing underlying support, speech improvement, promotion of oral hygiene, and for esthetic reasons. Crowns, inlays, outlays, bridges, and veneers are examples of fixed prosthodontics. The two categories of removable prosthodontics are partial dentures, which replace one or more teeth in an arch, and complete or full dentures, which take the place of all teeth in one arch. Partial dentures are held in place by underlying tissues and other teeth, while full dentures are supported by gingival and oral mucosal tissues, alveolar ridges and the hard palate.

## MAINTENANCE OF DENTAL PROSTHESES

**Fixed prostheses** are maintained by brushing and flossing. Toothbrushes selected should be soft, multi-tufted, and small enough to access all areas. Bridges can be cleaned by using a bridge threader to insert dental floss underneath. Interproximal brushes and tips are also available. Dental implants, which are titanium devices or screws that fuse with bone tissue by bonding (osseointegration), should be brushed with a similar type of brush and a specialized type of floss that is wider and designed to be wrapped around the implant (such as Proxi-Floss). Other maintenance measures include use of a plastic interproximal brush, water irrigators for plaque and debris removal, antimicrobial rinses, and a variety of plastic cleaning instruments. Removable prostheses or dentures are brushed with a special denture toothbrush and mild soap or toothpaste. Tissue under the denture should also be brushed. Dentures are removed and placed in cleaning agents to get rid of stains. Orthodontic devices should be maintained with specially designed toothbrushes, water irrigation, and an interproximal brush.

## CUSTOM TRAY

### CRITERIA

A **custom tray** is fabricated to make an accurate impression. Therefore, the tray must be durable enough to hold the material during positioning and removal. It should be smoothed and shaped to the patient's arch. Ideally, it should allow the impression material to fill with consistent thickness in all regions of the arch. The tray should be adaptable to any type of dentition, from an edentulous condition to full dentition, and any other type of unusual area. Trays that have stops in the spacer to grip the impression material are a good design and provide greater accuracy for the impression.

## MATERIALS

**Custom trays** are made from acrylic, resin, or a thermoplastic substance:

- *Self-curing acrylic tray resin* - This system combines a polymer powder with a liquid catalyst or monomer, initiating polymerization and exothermic release of heat. Complete setting to a very hard state takes about a day.
- *Light-cured acrylic tray resin* - Similar to self-curing acrylic, but remains malleable until a special curing light is activated, which initiates the polymerization and sets much faster.
- *Vacuum-formed custom trays* - These use heavy, stiff sheets of plastic resin. The resin is hung within a special unit and heated until soft. The sheet is then released onto the model, as vacuum pressure is applied.
- *Thermoplastic materials* - Beads or buttons are softened and made pliant through exposure to heat, usually warm water. After shaping, hardening occurs as heat disperses.

## OUTLINING MARGINS AND PREPARING CASTS

When **outlining the margins and preparing the cast** for a custom tray, first the dental assistant adapts a working plaster or stone cast. The assistant draws a blue line in the deepest area of the entire margin. The assistant draws a red line for wax spacer placement 1 to 2 mm above the blue line. The red mark corresponds to about 2 to 3 mm below the tooth margin or above the lowest point of the vestibule, if edentulous. Spacers are made of pink baseplate wax, a special molding material, or wet paper towels. The assistant plugs any recessed undercuts in the model. The spacer material is heated, shaped, and trimmed to the red line with a laboratory knife. Stops or holes are cut at intervals on the top edges of the spacer to permit impression material through. The assistant drapes the top of the spacer with aluminum foil, if self-cured resin is being used to dissipate heat and facilitate removal of wax at the end of the procedure. Sometimes, the assistant paints a separating material over the spacer.

## MIXING RESIN AND CONTOURING SELF-CURED ACRYLIC RESIN CUSTOM TRAYS

The dental assistant mixes the **self-curing resin** components, the powder polymer and the liquid catalyst, in a wax-lined paper cup with a wooden tongue blade, until the mixture is uniform. Follow the directions from the manufacturer. The initial set or polymerization takes about 2 to 3 minutes. Apply petroleum jelly to the palms and the cast. The dental assistant takes the malleable resin and manipulates it into a doughy patty or roll for a maxillary or mandibular arch. A little is reserved to make a handle later. The resin patty or roll is inserted over and extending slightly beyond (1 to 2 mm) the wax spacer. For the maxillary tray, this means inclusion of the palatal area. The assistant manually contours it with a rolled edge. Use of the laboratory knife is permitted, but less desirable. The handle material is molded and attached to the front of the tray, near the midline, using a drop of the monomer catalyst liquid.

## MAKING VACUUM-FORMED ACRYLIC RESIN CUSTOM TRAYS

The dental assistant prepares the previously-made cast by immersing it in warm water for up to 30 minutes to remove surface air bubbles. Add spacers, if specified. Outline the outer margin. Place the cast on a **vacuum-forming unit** with a platform. Secure the unit between two frames with acrylic resin sheets. These hang above the platform. One of the frames contains a heating element. Turn it on to cause the resin sheet to droop downward. When the resin hangs down about an inch, the operator pulls the frames down over the cast, using the handles on the sides. Activate the vacuum right after the resin drops over the cast. Turn the heat off. Keep the vacuum on for a minute or two. Once the tray cools, take it off the frame. Release it from the model, and trim it to the preferred form with a laboratory scissors. Cut a handle and attach it using a torch. Clean, disinfect and label the tray.

## FINISHING SELF-CURED ACRYLIC RESIN CUSTOM TRAYS

The procedure for **finishing a self-cured acrylic resin custom tray** is as follows:

- Don safety glasses.
- Remove the custom tray from the model and wax spacer after 8 to 10 minutes of setting.
- Remove the wax by melting or using a spatula, hot water, and a toothbrush.
- Trim the outside edges of the tray later, using an acrylic burr.
- Ensure the material is completely set (about 30 minutes).
- Clean disinfect, and label the tray.
- Before taking the impression, paint two thin coats of impression adhesive onto the inside of the tray and along the margins.
- Further secure the impression material by making holes in the tray with a round burr.

## DENTAL BLEACHING TRAY

Teeth whitening is the most common cosmetic dentistry procedure performed. There are several home products and methods for whitening the teeth, but in-office teeth whitening is the generally considered the safest and most effective method. The components of the **dental bleaching tray** will vary depending upon the manufacturer, but generally, the following supplies will be included:

- *Cheek retractor:* Holds the mouth open and cheeks away from the teeth to expose the teeth that are visible during smiling.
- *Liquid rubber dam or hardening resin:* Brushed onto the gum tissue to prevent irritation.
- *Bleaching gel:* This is a hydrogen peroxide-based gel that is applied to the teeth for 15 to 30 minutes. This is rinsed off and reapplied at least one more time for another 15 to 30 minutes.
- *Light:* Some products include a light that is used to illuminate the treated teeth during the whitening process. It is unclear whether this step increases the outcome of the whitening process.
- *Whitening outcome measure:* This measures the shade change to compare the color of the treated teeth before and after the procedure.

## POURING ALGINATE IMPRESSIONS FOR STUDY MODELS

The dental assistant makes the **study model**. Mix the plaster and pour it into the alginate impression. Hold the alginate impression over a vibrator on low or medium speed while the plaster is added, starting at the back of one side of the arch. The plaster should stream down the back of the impression. Add more plaster until it flows toward the front teeth to the other arch and out the other end, thus permeating the anatomical part of the model. Take the impression off the vibrator and pack the rest of the impression with plaster. Briefly vibrate the impression again for amalgamation. This is the anatomic portion of the model. If an art portion is to be added, the surface should retain small drops of plaster.

## ART PORTION OF PLASTER STUDY MODELS

The dental assistant is responsible for preparing the **art portion of the study model**. Pour the anatomical portion of the study model and set it for 5 to 10 minutes. Clean the flexible rubber or disposable bowl to prepare it for mixing more plaster. The ratio of water to powder for the art portion is 40 mL per 100 grams of powder (thicker than the 50 mL/100gm used for the anatomical portion). Use a spatula to put the mixture on a glass slab or paper towel, creating a base. Turn the anatomical part of the model over onto the base and position it so that the tray handle is parallel to the slab or paper. Scoop surplus plaster along the edges to fill gaps. This is the two-pour method.

The art portion can also be poured right after the anatomical part is filled by a single-pour technique. The model is allowed to set for 40 to 60 minutes, plaster on the outside of the tray is cut off with a laboratory knife, and the model is separated from the impression by holding the tray and lifting upwards.

## ARTICULATOR

**Articulators** are frames symbolizing the jaws. They are attached to study models to keep the models in occlusion and to move them. They are useful for examination of malocclusion. One of the most common types is the Stephan articulator, which is designed to demonstrate both up-and-down and sideways movements. It has hinges corresponding to the temporomandibular joints. A wax bite is placed temporarily to determine correct occlusion. The base of each model is scored, and then they are connected to bows on the device with additional impression plaster.

## POURING ALGINATE IMPRESSIONS WITH PLASTER

When **pouring an alginate impression with plaster**, the dental assistant makes the impression. Measure 50 ml of room temperature water into a flexible mixing bowl. Weigh 100 grams of plaster into another flexible bowl. Transfer the powder into the bowl with the water and let it dissolve. This makes a Type II model or laboratory plaster. Blend the particles with a metal spatula for about a minute. Press and rotate the bowl on a vibrator platform for several minutes, set at low to medium speed. This process introduces air bubbles that form to the top of the mixture. The desired consistency is creamy and smooth, but thick enough to remain in position.

## TRIMMING DIAGNOSTIC CASTS OR STUDY MODELS

When **trimming diagnostic casts or study models**, first don safety glasses. Wet the dry models in flexible mixing bowls. Ensure the base is parallel to the counter and occlusal plane. If not, trim it with the model trimmer. Apply even pressure on the trimming wheel, while supporting the hands on the trimmer table. Set the maxillary and mandibular models together in occlusion to examine further for parallelism. Once the two are parallel, draw a pencil line behind the retromolar area on the model. Trim the back of the model off perpendicular to the base. Reposition the two models in occlusion. Hold the two halves in place and cut off the untrimmed model at a right angle to its base, at the same spot as the opposing model. Draw lines as guides for trimming off the side areas, anterior cuts, and the heel portion. Trim the tongue area with a laboratory knife. Plaster fills the holes. Smooth with wet sandpaper. Apply model gloss. Polish the model and label it.

## SIDE TRIMMING

For **side trimming**, mark lines and make cuts on both models about 5 mm from and parallel to a line between the edge of the model and center of the premolars for the mandible, or the cuspids for the maxilla. Make anterior cuts on the maxillary model along a line from the midline to the area between the canine and cuspid on each quadrant. The line may need to be protruded outward, if teeth are in the way. For the mandibular model, make the anterior cuts back to each cuspid area in a more curved fashion. Heel cuts are small trimmed edges in the back on either side of each model that extend toward the center of the back.

## TRIMMED DIAGNOSTIC CAST OR STUDY MODEL

**Diagnostic casts** are shown to the patient to explain treatment. They should be *trimmed to specifications* and *look professionally prepared.* Approximately two-thirds of the model should be the anatomical portion (1 inch) and the other third the art portion or base (½ inch), for a total depth of 1½ inches. Displayed in occlusion, the total height should be 3 inches. Each model should be *symmetrically cut*, using the angles described elsewhere. Casts placed in occlusion should be capable of maintaining that relationship when placed on their ends together. If they fall apart, they are not trimmed properly.

## DENTAL LABORATORY PRESCRIPTION FORM

The **dental laboratory prescription form** is used to communicate to the dental laboratory exactly what restorative prosthetic is needed. A generic order or a specific form supplied by the dental laboratory should be used for accurate ordering. The order should be very specific in order for the finished product to be accurate. The dentist and the office staff should be familiar with the components necessary for creation of an accurate prosthesis and a positive outcome for the patient. Components to include on the dental laboratory prescription form are:

- Patient information: Name, age, gender, occupation, and lifestyle.
- Date of the request.
- Detailed description of the prosthetic needed.
- Specific materials and composition to be used – Acrylic, metal, ceramic, etc.
- Shade using a number and specific guide for instruction.
- Desired occlusion: Include accurate casts and the occlusal record. Dental photos may be included for accurate visualization of what type of prosthesis will be necessary.
- Desired turnaround time: An estimate should be given to the patient based on experience with the dental laboratory and their normal turnaround time for different types of prostheses.

# CDA Practice Test

Want to take this practice test in an online interactive format?
Check out the bonus page, which includes interactive practice questions and much more: **https://www.mometrix.com/bonus948/danbgc**

SCAN HERE

**1. Which of the following is not located within the oral cavity?**
   a. Hard palate
   b. Frenum
   c. Gingiva
   d. Pterygoid process

**2. How often should a patient be asked to update their medical and dental history?**
   a. At every visit
   b. Every 6 months
   c. Annually
   d. Only when something changes

**3. Which of the following would be least likely to be found on the clinical examination form?**
   a. Temporomandibular joint (TMJ) evaluation
   b. Dates of loss of primary teeth
   c. Dates of tooth extractions
   d. Information on crowns or bridge work

**4. Which of the following vital signs would be cause for concern during dental treatment?**
   a. Blood pressure of 140/90 mm Hg
   b. Respiratory rate of 18 breaths per minute
   c. Pulse of 70 beats per minute in an adult
   d. Oral temperature of 99 °F

**5. According to the Universal Numbering System, where is tooth 21 located?**
   a. Upper right cuspid
   b. Lower right lateral incisor
   c. Upper left 2nd molar
   d. Lower left 1st bicuspid

**6. In the positioning of the dental assistant for four-handed dentistry, which of the following is not recommended?**
   a. Eye level is positioned 4 to 6 inches above the dentist's eye level
   b. Feet placed on the foot ring or base of the stool and the stool is positioned close to the dental chair
   c. Legs are together, seating position is close to the back of the stool, feet planted firmly on the floor
   d. Stool positioned close to the dental chair with legs parallel to the dental chair

**7. What is the name of the right-handed operating zone from 4 o'clock to 7 o'clock?**

a. Operator's zone
b. Transfer zone
c. Assistant's zone
d. Static zone

**8. What is the name of the instrument that includes the following types: straight, binangle, Wedelstaedt, and angle-former?**

a. Excavator
b. Hatchet
c. Gingival trimmer
d. Chisel

**9. What type of instrument is a burnisher?**

a. Restorative
b. Accessory
c. Basic
d. Hand cutting

**10. A patient undergoing a procedure of approximately 30 minutes will most likely require which of the following types of anesthetics?**

a. Bupivacaine
b. Prilocaine HCl block
c. Novocain
d. Lidocaine HCl

**11. What type of procedure would include the following instruments: matrix set up, burs, saliva ejector, HVE, dental dam setup, and local anesthetic set up?**

a. Extraction
b. Root canal
c. Class II amalgam restoration
d. Incision and drainage

**12. What type of instrument is used to remove enamel during the placement of a veneer?**

a. Condenser
b. Diamond bur
c. Evacuator
d. Carver

**13. What type of instrument is used by the dentist to lower the height of the tooth during preparation for a crown?**

a. Bevel instrument
b. Carver
c. High-speed handpiece
d. Ultrasonic handpiece

**14. The air abrasion handpiece is least likely to be used in which of the following procedures?**

    a. Gingival retraction
    b. External stain removal
    c. Sealants
    d. Class II preparations

**15. Which of the following supplies would most likely NOT be used for taking a mandibular preliminary impression?**

    a. Wide-blade spatula
    b. Biohazard bag
    c. Alginate measure scoop
    d. Polycarboxylate

**16. Which of the following is NOT true regarding the application of topical fluoride foam?**

    a. Patients should be instructed not to swallow the fluoride
    b. Patients may eat or drink right away
    c. The teeth should be dry before the fluoride foam is applied
    d. A double arch tray may be used to apply fluoride to both arches at the same time

**17. The vitality test is used to measure the health of:**

    a. enamel.
    b. dentin.
    c. pulp.
    d. root.

**18. When applying a topical anesthetic ointment in preparation for the dentist to give an injection, what is the longest length of time the topical ointment will provide optimal effectiveness?**

    a. 1 minute
    b. 2 minutes
    c. 5 minutes
    d. 7 minutes

**19. Which of the following is TRUE about the administration of nitrous oxide and oxygen ($N_2O/O_2$)?**

    a. The patient should be encourage to mouth breathe in order to maximize the effectiveness of $N_2O/O_2$
    b. Once the dosage is determined for $N_2O/O_2$, the same dosage can be used at subsequent dental visits
    c. The $N_2O/O_2$ procedure should end with the administration of 100% pure oxygen for at least an hour
    d. Administration of $N_2O/O_2$ should begin with 100% pure oxygen

**20. When assisting with the delivery of a partial denture, which of the following is NOT something a dental assistant would be responsible for?**

 a. Adjusting the tension on the retainer
 b. Disinfecting the prosthesis before it is placed in the patient's mouth
 c. Placing articulating paper in the patient's mouth in order to check the occlusion
 d. Polishing the prosthesis before delivering to patient for instruction on use

**21. When assisting with root canal therapy, what is the first instrument the dentist will need to enter the coronal portion of the tooth?**

 a. Carbide round bur
 b. Endodontic explorer
 c. Reamer files
 d. Dental broach

**22. When assisting with a scaling procedure for periodontal debridement, what instrument is used by the dentist to remove supragingival and subgingival calculus?**

 a. Prophy angle
 b. Kirkland knife
 c. Gracey curette
 d. Periotome

**23. Which of the following statements would be the most effective in communicating with an apprehensive patient?**

 a. The next sound you hear will be the drill.
 b. We are preparing the tooth for restoration.
 c. You will likely feel a little pain initially but it will subside once the anesthetic kicks in.
 d. I am applying a topical anesthetic before the dentist comes in to give you the shot.

**24. What is the least effective strategy a dental assistant can take to assist a hearing-impaired patient in understanding instructions?**

 a. Remove mask before speaking to allow patient to see lips
 b. Try to reduce other noise in the area when trying to communicate with the patient
 c. Use written illustrations and handouts for the patient to read
 d. Speak very loudly so the patient can hear you better

**25. Which of the following may be contraindicated in a patient with severe hypertension?**

 a. Fluoride
 b. Nitrous oxide
 c. Levonordefrin
 d. Lidocaine

**26. Which of the following would not be the first choice for managing a reluctant child during a routine cleaning appointment?**

 a. Ask the child to hold and assist with the saliva ejector
 b. Involve the child in the procedure such as selecting the flavor of fluoride or toothpaste
 c. Use a papoose board
 d. Allow the parent to stay in the room to help keep the child calm

**27. A patient who has had a heart transplant comes in for a dental procedure. He has a history of a penicillin allergy but needs to take prophylactic antibiotics prior to the procedure. Which antibiotic would most likely be prescribed?**

    a. Amoxicillin
    b. Erythromycin
    c. Ampicillin
    d. Cephalexin

**28. Which of the following dental products would NOT be used for a final impression?**

    a. Alginate
    b. Polysulfide
    c. Polyether
    d. Silicone

**29. Which of the following is the last step in the preparation and application of a composite resin material?**

    a. Have the liquid bonding resin available for use by the dentist
    b. Use the cure light
    c. Apply final carving touches
    d. Select the appropriate shade of composite

**30. What is the proper ratio for mixing a noneugenol dressing?**

    a. 1 part base to 3 parts accelerator materials
    b. 1 part accelerator to 3 parts base materials
    c. 2 parts base to 1 part accelerator materials
    d. Equal parts base and accelerator materials

**31. Which type of polishing agent is the best choice for polishing porcelain?**

    a. Sapphire polishing paste
    b. Aluminum oxide paste
    c. Silex
    d. Fluoride paste

**32. Which of the following statements is false concerning light-cured sealant application?**

    a. Poor sealant retention on the tooth surface may be due to contamination of the sealant with saliva during application.
    b. Dental dams or cotton rolls will help to maintain a dry field when applying sealants.
    c. Shining the curing light for 30 seconds will be the appropriate length of time to cure all surfaces that have been sealed.
    d. Use floss to make sure there is no sealant in contact with the interproximal area of the teeth.

**33. What type of product is optimal for use in study models for the fabrication of a dental bridge?**

    a. Dental stone
    b. Plaster of Paris
    c. Alginate
    d. Densite

**34. What would be the appropriate type of wax to select for setting denture teeth?**

    a.  Casting wax

    b.  Baseplate wax

    c.  Inlay casting wax

    d.  Utility wax

**35. All of the following are true about plaque formation except:**

    a.  the bacteria responsible for plaque formation are mutans streptococci and lactobacilli.

    b.  proper brushing and flossing can remove plaque.

    c.  the action of saliva will remove any remaining plaque following flossing.

    d.  potatoes and pasta promote plaque formation.

**36. What is the effect of chronic overexposure to fluoride?**

    a.  Nausea

    b.  Diarrhea

    c.  Stomatitis

    d.  Fluorosis

**37. Which of the following vitamins or minerals is not directly related to tooth formation?**

    a.  Vitamin D

    b.  Phosphorus

    c.  Folic acid

    d.  Magnesium

**38. Which of the following statements would NOT be a recommendation given to parents to help reduce the risk of cavity formation in their 8-year-old child?**

    a.  Drink juice or water instead of soda

    b.  Avoid sticky foods such as raisins, dried fruits, granola bars, caramel, Skittles, and jelly beans

    c.  Offer cheese as a snack or part of a meal

    d.  Chew gum sweetened with xylitol.

**39. A patient has finished his first visit for crown placement. The provisional coverage has been placed on the tooth in preparation for the crown placement. All of the following are appropriate instructions to the patient EXCEPT:**

    a.  avoid sticky foods.

    b.  floss carefully and gently slide the floss between the temporary crown and the adjacent tooth.

    c.  be careful chewing in the area of the provisional coverage to prevent damage from occurring to the temporary crown.

    d.  if the temporary crown comes off, it is acceptable to wait until the next appointment to inform the dentist.

**40. Which of the following is used most frequently in a medical emergency?**

    a.  Oxygen

    b.  Spirits of ammonia

    c.  EpiPen

    d.  Nitroglycerin

**41. A pregnant patient receiving dental treatment may experience which of the following after sitting up quickly in the chair?**

    a.  Postural hypertension
    b.  Hypoglycemia
    c.  Postural hypotension
    d.  Syncope

**42. A patient experiencing difficulty speaking, paralysis, vision impairment, or sudden headache may be experiencing a(n):**

    a.  myocardial infarction.
    b.  migraine.
    c.  cerebrovascular accident.
    d.  seizure.

**43. A patient with type 1 diabetes is receiving dental care. The patient is complaining of dry mouth and a headache. You notice a fruity, acetone odor on the patient's breath. What is the appropriate action?**

    a.  Provide a source of concentrated sugar such as orange juice or a sugar packet to help raise blood sugar level.
    b.  You determine that the patient has skipped the morning insulin dose and assist the patient with insulin administration
    c.  Call 911 immediately
    d.  Call the patient's emergency contact

**44. You observe creamy white lesions that look like cottage cheese on the tongue and cheeks of one of your patients. This patient likely has:**

    a.  herpes zoster.
    b.  herpes simplex.
    c.  lichen planus.
    d.  oral candidiasis.

**45. Dental office employees may be at risk for certain types of occupational exposures to certain diseases. What type of hepatitis vaccination is required by OSHA to be offered to these employees within 10 days of initial job assignment?**

    a.  Hepatitis A
    b.  Hepatitis B
    c.  Hepatitis C
    d.  Hepatitis D

**46. What method for ordering supplies would be used to obtain the best discount on dental supplies while having to stock only a part of the order at any one time?**

    a.  Automatic shipments
    b.  Quantity purchase rate
    c.  Reorder quantity
    d.  Reorder point

**47. What type of plan is necessary to assist with repairs for frequently used equipment in a dental office?**

    a. Manufacturer warranty
    b. Service contract
    c. Equipment records including serial number and model
    d. Extended warranty

**48. What is the term used to describe the amount of money that must be paid toward the cost of dental treatment before insurance benefits will be activated?**

    a. Deductible
    b. Copayment
    c. Benefit eligibility
    d. Customary fee

**49. Which of the following is not true about the state Dental Practice Act?**

    a. The act provides requirements for licensure and renewal of licenses.
    b. It specifies the duties that may be performed by a dental assistant or a dental hygienist.
    c. It specifies regulations and requirements surrounding infection control and radiation use.
    d. The act is the same from state to state but is enforced by individual state dental boards

**50. What is the name of the law that requires dental offices to have a written policy regarding patient privacy?**

    a. OSHA
    b. Privacy Act of 1986
    c. HIPAA
    d. Dental Practice Act

# Answer Key and Explanations

**1. D:** The pterygoid process is located in the skull but not within the oral cavity. The oral cavity is the area located within the mouth. The lips are the entrance to the oral cavity. Parts of the oral cavity include the vestibule and the labial, which includes the frenum. It also includes the gingival or gums. The oral cavity proper refers to the area within the oral cavity that can be found inside of the dental arches. It includes the hard and soft palates, the tongue, taste buds, and teeth. The uvula is located within the oral cavity and is part of the soft palate.

**2. A:** The medical/dental health history is a very important part of a patient's dental record. The medical history provides information on both current and long-term conditions that may affect dental treatment, medication use, allergies, and any other pertinent information. The dental history gathers information about previous dental treatments and experiences, as well as dental habits. It is very important to ask the patient at each visit if there is any change in medical or dental history because certain changes may impact dental treatment. This could be a new allergy to an antibiotic, pregnancy, or development of heart disease. Any change should be noted as it may be important.

**3. B:** The clinical examination form is one of the most important forms in the patient's dental record. It provides very detailed information on past dental treatment, including location and dates of fillings, extractions, and crown and bridge work and other types of dental prostheses. The form also details examination of the oral cavity, soft tissue, overall oral hygiene, and condition of gums. Assessment of temporomandibular joint disorder is recorded here as well. Present and future planned examination should be recorded on this form. Any patient education is also documented on the clinical examination form.

**4. A:** Dental procedures may affect a person's vital signs. It is important to know how to check vital signs when needed in order to help make an assessment of whether to continue treatment. The 4 vital signs are temperature, pulse, respiration, and blood pressure. A normal oral temperature can range from 97.6 to 99 °F. An increased temperature may indicate an infection and dental treatment may need to be postponed. A normal pulse or heart rate for an adult is 60-100 beats per minute at rest and 70-120 beats per minute for a child. A normal respiratory rate is 10-20 breaths per minute for an adult and 18-30 breaths per minute for a child or teen. Increases in pulse or respiratory rate may reflect stress, age, medications, or other reasons. A normal blood pressure is a systolic reading less than 120 mm Hg and a diastolic less than 80 mm Hg. Elevated blood pressure at the time of a dental exam may also require postponement.

**5. D:** There are three systems for numbering teeth. The Universal Numbering System is most commonly used in the United States. The mouth is viewed from the perspective of looking into the patient's mouth so when referring to the right or left, this should correspond to the patient's right or left. The mouth is divided into the following 4 quadrants: upper left, upper right, lower right, and lower left. The teeth are numbered starting with the upper right 3rd molar and ending with the lower right 3rd molar. The 3rd molars are teeth numbers 1, 16, 17, and 32. The 2nd molars are 2, 15, 18, and 31. The 1st molars are 3, 14, 19, and 30. The 2nd bicuspids are 4, 13, 20, and 29. The 1st bicuspids are 5, 12, 21, and 28. The cuspids are 6, 11, 22, and 27. The lateral incisors are 7, 10, 23, and 26, and the central incisors are 8, 9, 24, and 25. Wisdom teeth are considered 1, 16, 17, and 32.

**6. C:** Proper positioning for the dental assistant is extremely important. A specialized stool is used to help provide comfort and promote easy mobility while protecting against unnecessary strain to the upper body. The dental assistant should be seated towards the back of the stool, close to the

**146**

dental chair, and legs should be parallel with the dental chair. The feet should rest on the bottom of the stool such as the foot ring. The eye level of the dental assistant should be 4-6 inches above that of the dentist or other type of operator such as dental hygienist.

**7. B:** Operating zones were developed as a way to provide an efficient working zone that is comfortable and safe for the dental assistant and the operator (usually a dentist but could also be a hygienist). The operating zone is based on a clock concept where the patient's head is positioned at 12 o'clock. The transfer zone for a right-handed person is 4 o'clock to 7 o'clock. This is the zone where the dental assistant and dentist give instruments or materials to one another above the patient's chest. The operator's zone for a right-handed person is between 7 o'clock and 12 o'clock. The assistant's zone is considered between 2 and 4 o'clock for a right-handed person. The static zone is between 10 and 12 o'clock and is located behind the patient. If the proper zones are observed by each individual, the chance of bumping into each other is minimized.

**8. D:** Hand-cutting instruments are used to allow the dentist to easily remove the parts of the tooth that are decayed. These instruments are positioned next to the basic setup on the tray. Types of hand-cutting instruments include the excavator, hoe, chisel, hatchet, and gingival margin trimmer. Many types of chisels are available, all with a slightly different function. Straight, binangle, Wedelstaedt, and angle-former are all types of chisels. Chisels are used to get through the enamel part of the tooth or to make straight lines. Most dentists will have their personal preference as to what type of chisels they use most often.

**9. A:** Restorative instruments are used in the placement of dental materials such as amalgam within the anatomy of the tooth. These instruments also help to shape the dental material into the correct position on the tooth. Types of restorative instruments include amalgam carrier, condensers, burnisher, carvers, composite placement instrument, and the Woodson. A burnisher is used for smoothing the surface after the amalgam is placed. A carver is used to take away any excess dental material or to make the appropriate indentations in the amalgam to fit the tooth's anatomy before it hardens. A condenser is used to push the dental material into the tooth so it is appropriately packed. The Woodson is the tool used for bringing the dental materials over to the tooth.

**10. D:** The most commonly used anesthetic in dentistry is lidocaine HCl. It is a type of short-duration anesthetic used for procedures expecting to last approximately 30 minutes. For procedures that will last about an hour, an intermediate-duration anesthetic will most likely be selected by the dentist. This would include lidocaine with epinephrine, mepivacaine with epinephrine, prilocaine HCl (with and without epinephrine), and articaine with epinephrine. Long-duration anesthetic such as bupivacaine with epinephrine is used for procedures that will last 90 minutes or more. Procaine (*Novocain*) is not used as frequently as a short-duration anesthetic since the introduction of lidocaine.

**11. C:** A Class II amalgam restoration includes restorative tray containing basic setup, composite placement instrument, condensers, burnishers, carvers, and articulating paper holder. It also includes the setups for local anesthesia, dental dam, and matrix. High-volume oral evacuator (HVE) and saliva ejector are also included. Dental liners, base sealers, and bonding agents, as well as prefilled amalgam capsules, would be on the tray. The dental assistant would provide assistance to the dentist in the administration of the local anesthetic. During the preparation of the tooth for the restoration, the dental assistant would use the HVE and air/water syringes as needed to keep the area clear for the dentist to work. The dental assistant would mix the amalgam using the amalgamator and assist in the transfer of amalgam to the dentist. Assistance would also be provided as the amalgam is shaped, condensed, carved, and adjusted.

**12. B:** A veneer is a coating of tooth-colored material (to match the rest of the teeth) over a tooth that has been discolored, darkened, eroded, or chipped. Veneers are also used to help with alignment and lengthening. A diamond bur is used by the dentist to remove a specified amount of enamel in order to prepare the tooth for the placement of the veneer. The surrounding teeth are protected with celluloid matrix strips before the dental materials are applied. The dental assistant may help with transferring tools, curing the veneer, and communicating with the patient.

**13. C:** Placement of a crown typically takes 2 dental visits. The first visit involves selecting the proper shade for the crown, taking initial impressions, preparing the tooth, and taking final impressions. Rotary tools such as the low- or high-speed handpiece are used to lower the actual height of the tooth as well as to properly contour the tooth so the crown will fit over the tooth and remain the same size as the original tooth. The first visit also includes placement of a temporary crown to protect the area being worked on. The second visit will include the actual placement of the crown for proper fit and cementing into place.

**14. A:** The air abrasion unit has been in use since the 1940s. The air abrasion handpiece is used for cavities and stain removal. Aluminum oxide particles are delivered via a high-pressure delivery system. This procedure removes enamel, stains, and other types of dental material without damaging the tooth. Local anesthesia is not required and is a gentler way of delivering care to patients. The air abrasion handpiece is especially effective when used for placement of sealants, access for endodontic procedures, crown margins, preparation of tooth for crown placement, and preparation of tooth for Class I through VI restoration.

**15. D:** Alginate powder is the type of dental material used for taking mandibular or maxillary impressions. Polycarboxylate is a type of cement used for other dental procedures. Other equipment required for taking impressions is the scoop and water measure that are provided by the manufacturer for preparing the alginate. Water that is at room temperature should be available. The powder is mixed in a rubber bowl using a wide-blade spatula. The material is then spread onto the sterile impression tray and pressed upon with the spatula in order to remove air bubbles that may interfere with the quality of the impression.

**16. B:** Fluoride is a mineral that helps keep teeth healthy by preventing tooth decay. Some water supplies are fluoridated; however, patients who do not have fluoridated water will require some form of fluoride supplements. Professionally applied fluoride is often indicated for some children. Fluoride gels or foam are commonly used for this purpose. The fluoride is placed in the disposable tray. The patient must be seated in an upright position to help prevent fluoride from accidently being swallowed. The teeth are dried using the air-water syringe. The tray is put into the mouth and the patient is instructed to bite down. The fluoride is squeezed over the teeth. The saliva ejector is used to clean out the saliva so the fluoride is not swallowed. After the appropriate application time, the saliva ejector is used to remove the saliva and fluoride. The patient should not rinse the mouth or eat or drink anything for at least 30 minutes in order to maximize the effectiveness of the fluoride treatment.

**17. C:** The vitality test in dentistry is used to evaluate the health of the pulp, which is the tissue or nerve located inside the tooth. This test can provide valuable information for diagnostic and treatment planning purposes. The vitality test checks to see if there is a nerve issue. This is typically done on teeth that have undergone some sort of trauma. A root canal removes the pulp from the tooth, so the vitality test would provide no information for this tooth. The following techniques can be used to check the pulp: palpation of the area above the root, apply cold or heat to the tooth, or use the electric pulp test (EPT). The dental assistant would typically assist the dentist with this procedure and record results of the testing.

**18. B:** Topical anesthetics are used before the injection is given to numb the nerve endings in the area of the injection site. Multiple forms of topical anesthetics include ointments, spray, patches, and liquids. The topical patch is the fastest acting agent at approximately 10 seconds; the other agents will start to work in approximately 15-30 seconds. The topical ointment is applied using a cotton tip applicator. The area where the injection will be given should be gently dried using cotton gauze. The ointment should be applied just below the injection site. The applicator should remain in place for at least 15-30 seconds and until the dentist is ready to give the injection. The longest length of time that the numbing effect will be felt is usually around 1-2 minutes.

**19. D:** Nitrous oxide/oxygen ($N_2O/O_2$) analgesia is also known as inhalation sedation. It has been in use since 1844. This type of sedation is administered through a nosepiece and is fast acting. $N_2O/O_2$ provides a very relaxing and good experience for the patient but can become habit forming if abused. A tightly fitting face mask should be used for administration and the patient should be instructed not to talk or breathe through the mouth to prevent nitrous oxide ($N_2O$) from escaping. The process starts with the administration of pure oxygen to establish the patient's tidal volume. $N_2O$ is then titrated to achieve appropriate results. The dosage of $N_2O$ can vary from one visit to the next; therefore, the dose must be reestablished each time. The $N_2O/O_2$ analgesia process should conclude with the administration of pure oxygen for approximately 3-5 minutes. The patient should be evaluated for the presence of headache, lethargy, or dizziness. If any of these symptoms are present, the patient should continue to receive 100% oxygen until the symptoms normalize.

**20. A:** The dental assistant will lead the patient into the dental chair. After the prosthesis is scrubbed and disinfected, the dentist will place it in the patient's mouth. The dentist examines the fit and use of the dentures. The dental assistant places articulating paper into the patient's mouth in order to check the occlusion or the contact between the upper and lower teeth. Pressure indicator paste is also used to check for pressure points on the tissue that touches the prosthesis. The dentist makes appropriate adjustments for the comfort of the patient, including adjustment of the tension. Finally, the partial denture is polished and then thoroughly cleaned and disinfected before being given to the patient. The patient is educated regarding proper use and care of the partial dentures.

**21. A:** Root canal therapy involves removing the dental pulp and replacing it with dental material. The dentist will need the carbide round bur to enter into the coronal part of the tooth to start the process of removing the decay and inner structure of the tooth. The next instrument will be the endodontic explorer and other intracanal instruments. These instruments may include endodontic spoon excavator, spreaders, and pluggers, which are used in the obturation of the canal. A Glick no. 1 instrument is used to place the temporary restorations. There are a variety of files, both hand and rotary operated, that will also be used within the pulpal cavity, such as the K-type file, Hedstrom file, Reamer file, and broaches.

**22. C:** Periodontics is the treatment of diseases pertaining to tissues within the mouth, such as the gums. A periodontal exam is much like a regular dental exam, which includes a medical and dental history, x-rays, and oral examination. There are specialized instruments used for periodontal procedures, such as scaling, root planing, and periodontal surgery. Periodontal probes measure the depth of periodontal pockets and periodontal explorers are used to find the location of calculus deposits on the supragingival or subgingival surfaces. Scaling is the removal of supragingival or subgingival calculus from teeth. Curettes are used to remove deposits on the subgingival and supragingival surfaces. Two types of curettes are the universal and the Gracey. Scalers are also used for this purpose and the main difference between curettes and scalers are the shape. Curettes are rounded and scalers have a pointed end. Root planing is the procedure that removes the remainder of the calculus and smoothes the surface to make cleaning of the area easier.

**23. B:** Dental fear or phobia is very real and how a patient is approached can make a big difference in future treatment. Verbal communication is very important. It is important to communicate with the patient in a way that he or she will understand. It is also important to make appropriate word choices to minimize the patient's reaction. Certain words, such as pain, shot, drill, or filling, may evoke fear or intimidation. Words that may be substituted include discomfort, anesthetic, prepare tooth, or restoration. These may be more effective. Nonverbal communication is also important. The patient is able to observe body language, so it is important to show a positive, stress-free image to the patient. This can be accomplished by breathing slowly and deeply, using calm facial expressions, and having an overall positive attitude. Good listening skills are also essential.

**24. D:** A patient with sensory deficits, such as hearing or sight, can be challenging but there are steps available to address issues. For the hearing-impaired patient, simply speaking loudly is not a viable option. The dental assistant may not be aware of the degree of hearing impairment and it may be intrusive to other patients. Better approaches would be to make sure the patient can see the mouth and lips when speaking and to speak clearly and enunciate each word. It is best to try to reduce the amount of additional noise in the room when trying to communicate, such as the suction machine or television or music. Simple, concise instructions should be provided, and illustrations or handouts should be used whenever possible. In some situations, a sign language interpreter may be needed.

**25. C:** Levonordefrin (*Neo-Cobefrin*) and epinephrine are vasoconstrictors that should be avoided in certain situations. A vasoconstrictor is a type of drug that causes the smooth muscles to constrict or narrow. This may cause undue strain on the heart or other organs. Patients with a history of severe hypertension, unstable angina, recent heart attacks or bypass surgery, or uncontrolled congestive heart failure should not receive a vasoconstrictor. Instead, an anesthetic without a vasoconstrictor should be used such as lidocaine or prilocaine HCl. Nitrous oxide can also be used. Another helpful consideration for patients with heart disease is to minimize the length of the appointment if possible, to avoid additional stress. Vital signs should be monitored and some patients may require supplemental oxygen during a procedure.

**26. C:** Developing a positive relationship with a child is very important in establishing good dental habits and a good attitude about dental visits. Many dentists will use the Frankl scale, which rates the child's behavior on a scale from 1 to 4 in order to track behavior over time. Simple steps can be taken to make the dental visit a pleasant experience. The child can be involved in the visit by holding the saliva ejector, choosing the flavor of toothpaste or fluoride, and helping select where to start the procedure. Explanations should be given to the child in simple terms, followed by showing the child what will be done and then doing exactly what you have told the child. Positive reinforcement is always helpful, such as a reward at the end of the visit. Parents can be allowed to stay in the room to help calm a patient but sometimes this can make the situation worse. A papoose board is not typically a choice during cleanings.

**27. B:** Certain patients will require short-term or prophylactic antibiotics when preparing for a dental procedure. These patients include those with artificial heart valves, history of endocarditis, heart transplant, and congenital heart disease. Forms of penicillin such as amoxicillin and ampicillin are commonly prescribed. Cephalosporins, such as cephalexin (*Keflex*), are antibiotics that are closely related to penicillin. Patients with an allergy to penicillin should not be prescribed antibiotics from either group. Antibiotics that could be substituted in this situation may be erythromycin or clindamycin. Some patients do not tolerate erythromycin and may show symptoms of nausea or abdominal distress. This should be monitored and an alternative drug should be prescribed by the dentist as needed.

**28. A:** Alginate is an irreversible hydrocolloid used to make preliminary impressions. Two types are available, normal set and fast set. The fast set can be used for patients with an extreme gag reflex or if there is only one person working to take the impression. Elastomeric materials are used to make final impressions. The available types include polyether, silicone, polysulfide, and polysiloxane. Each material is slightly different from the other. These materials have three forms: light, regular, or heavy bodied. The light bodied is used first followed by the heavy bodied. After the material has gone through initial set and final set, it is removed from the mouth. Final cure occurs between 1 and 24 hours. Properties include dimensional stability (the ability of the impression to stay intact after removal from the mouth), deformation (the ability of the impression to stay intact during removal from the mouth), and permanent deformation (the impression will remain in the shape after it changes).

**29. B:** Composite resins are more commonly used in dentistry for anterior teeth as well as some posterior teeth. Class I through V restorations can be completed with this product as well as the closing of diastema (space between front teeth) or restoration of abrasions or surface defects due to attrition or hypocalcification. The first step in the procedure for preparing and applying composite resin materials is to select the appropriate shade. Next the syringe is prepared and moved into the transfer zone for the dentist. The dentist applies the resin to the appropriate tooth and the curing light is then used for final setting of the resin. After the material is applied and set, there is a finishing and polishing stage. Finishing burs and any abrasive materials are contraindicated. A white stone or finishing diamond is used to gently reduce the resin followed by the use of diamond burs or other superfine burs to polish the resin. Polishing paste is used last to finish the process.

**30. D:** Noneugenol is the most commonly used dressing in periodontics. There are 2 parts to the dressing: the base material and the accelerator. Equal parts of each type of material should be mixed on a paper pad. Using a tongue depressor, both pastes should be mixed until they are evenly distributed and the color is consistent throughout the paste. The paste can be prevented from sticking to gloves by coating the gloves with saline. Once the noneugenol dressing is mixed, it should be used immediately. Exposure to warm temperatures will cause the material to set very quickly.

**31. A:** It is very important to take the time to select the appropriate polishing agent. Polishing material is made of abrasive materials and is available in different degrees of coarseness called grit. The higher the amount of grit, the more abrasive the agent is. All polishing agents remove some enamel but the end result is to select the agent that will cause the least amount of abrasion. Sapphire or diamond polishing paste is the appropriate selection to be used on porcelain surfaces. Aluminum oxide should be used on hybrid and resin composites. Silex is an abrasive agent and should only be selected for teeth with a moderate to heavy amount of staining. Zirconium silicate is an agent that is less abrasive to tooth enamel than other choices.

**32. C:** The sealant application process is very detailed. The surface of the tooth is first cleaned using a rubber cup and pumice or by air polishing the surface. Next, the enamel is etched using 37% phosphoric acid to allow the pores within the enamel to open up and accept the sealant material. Next, drying of the surface is extremely important. The presence of any moisture will cause the sealant to fail. A dental dam or cotton rolls can be used to maintain a dry field around the area. Light-cured sealants require the use of a curing light to cure or set the sealant. The light is shone on the surface for 20 seconds. Each surface that has received sealant application must be cured separately. Dental floss should be used to make sure sealant has not entered into the interproximal spaces. After the sealant application, the patient's bite should be checked using articulating paper.

**33. D:** Gypsum is the material that is used to make dental models used for orthodontic treatment, custom tray development, prosthetic devices, and the production of custom mouth guards. There are 3 forms of gypsum used. Densite (also known as improved dental stone) is used for the fabrication of dental bridges, crowns, or indirect restoration. Dental stone is used for the production of dentures. Plaster of Paris or model plaster is used for making preliminary impressions for orthodontic treatment. Water is required for nuclei of crystallization to occur. This promotes the growth of crystals during the setting process to provide strength and hardness to the final mold product. The ratio of water to powder is extremely important and requires careful measurement. For model plaster, the ratio is 100 g of plaster to 45-50 mL of water. For dental stone, the ratio is 100 g of powder to 30-32 mL of water, and for Densite, the ratio is 100 g of powder to 19-24 mL of water.

**34. B:** Dental wax is made from natural products including beeswax or fatty acids. It can also be made from synthetic materials to provide the necessary qualities needed for certain dental procedures. Each type of dental wax has a specific function in a dental laboratory. Baseplate wax is used for setting denture teeth. It is also used in initial arch form molds for the recording of the occlusal rim. Inlay casting wax is a harder type of wax used for producing a pattern of the indirect restoration from a model. Casting wax is used when concentrating on a single tooth for indirect restorations, a fixed bridge, or the metal portion of partial denture plate. Utility wax is used for comfort in orthodontic treatment by covering a bracket that may be irritating to gums during treatment. Boxing wax is used for in making preliminary impressions by surrounding the wall of the model to make a cleaner model without as much trimming required.

**35. C:** Plaque is a clear, sticky substance that sticks to teeth. Two types of bacteria are responsible for plaque formation: mutans streptococci and *Lactobacillus*. This type of bacteria can be transmitted from one person to another. Proper brushing and flossing can help to keep plaque under control but saliva alone is not strong enough to remove or control plaque formation. A diet that contains a high amount of fermentable carbohydrates will contribute to plaque formation. Foods such as potatoes, pasta, bread, and sugar are considered fermentable carbohydrates. This means that when this type of food is consumed, the bacteria begin to feed on this and produce a byproduct that is capable of penetrating the enamel, leading to caries.

**36. D:** Fluoride is a mineral that is often added to water supplies to help with dental health. It is also present in toothpaste and children receive fluoride treatments as part of routine dental exams. Fluoride is also present in many foods in small amounts. Fluoride is considered safe at low levels but chronic overexposure to fluoride can lead to fluorosis. This can be seen as mottling or an opaque area on the surfaces of the teeth. Severe fluorosis can lead to deep brown pits on the teeth that look like decay. Acute or short-term overexposure to fluoride can cause nausea, vomiting, diarrhea, and pain in the abdominal area. In severe cases of acute toxicity, convulsions, irregular heartbeat, and even coma can result.

**37. C:** The main vitamins and minerals that are involved in tooth formation are vitamin D, calcium, phosphorus, magnesium, and fluorine. Vitamins A, C, and E are also important for healthy gums. Sources of vitamin D include fortified milk, eggs, and fish. The body can also produce vitamin D with sun exposure. Vitamin D deficiency is becoming more and more common and has a significant impact on enamel formation, leading to an increase in cavities. Sources of calcium include dairy products, soy products, and green leafy vegetables. Sources of phosphorus include dairy products, meat, eggs, and whole grain products. Sources of magnesium include leafy green vegetables, nuts, grains, seafood, and bananas. Good nutrition is important to healthy teeth and gums. It is best for vitamins and minerals to be obtained through natural food sources instead of supplementation whenever possible. The exception is vitamin D, which may require over-the-counter supplementation with medical guidance.

**38. A:** Many food-related tips or suggestions can be offered to parents to help reduce the risk of cavity formation. Water is the best beverage to choose over juice or soda because these contain sugar. Milk also contains sugar but does provide other nutrients important to dental health. Sticky foods, such as raisins, dried fruits, or granola bars, or chewy candy, such as Skittles or jelly beans, are not good for teeth. If the child eats any of these foods, the teeth should be brushed right away. Foods that stay in a child's mouth for a prolonged period, such as lollipops or hard candies, should be avoided. Including cheese as part of a snack or meal is good for teeth as it helps to increase the amount of saliva produced, which helps to cleanse teeth. Crunchy fruits and vegetables are a good choice for children. The use of sugarless gum or gum sweetened with xylitol helps to reduce bacteria formation within the mouth and to produce saliva.

**39. D:** Placement of a crown typically takes 2 visits. The first visit includes selection of the appropriate shade for the crown, preliminary impressions, preparation of the tooth including core buildup and retention pins, and final impressions. The first visit also includes placement of the temporary crown or provisional coverage. It is very important for the patient to be aware of how important the provisional coverage is for the crown procedure. If any damage occurs to the temporary crown, it can negatively affect the final crown placement. If the temporary crown is damaged or dislodged, the dentist should be contacted immediately for replacement. Other instructions that should be given are to avoid sticky foods and to carefully chew in the area of the provisional coverage. Instruction on proper flossing should be provided. Floss should be gently slid between the temporary crown and the adjacent teeth below the contact to prevent damage from occurring. The second visit will include the cementing and finishing of the crown.

**40. A:** Oxygen is used most often in a medical emergency. It is required for any patient who has is unresponsive but still breathing and is absolutely necessary for a patient who has stopped breathing. Portable oxygen tanks should be readily available in the dental office should the need arise for oxygen administration. Other drugs that should be on hand include spirits of ammonia for trying to arouse someone who has fainted, an *EpiPen*, *Chlor-Trimeton*, and *Benadryl* for an allergic reaction, and nitroglycerin for angina pain. Albuterol is required for bronchospasms or asthma attacks and *Valium* for seizures. A source of rapidly absorbed sugar should be available, such as orange juice or sugar, for a hypoglycemic reaction. Methoxamine (*Vasoxyl*) should be available for issues with blood pressure and atropine should be available for bradycardia.

**41. C:** Postural hypotension is also known as orthostatic hypotension. It is a form of low blood pressure. This condition may occur when moving into an upright position too quickly. The person may experience dizziness, lightheadedness, nausea, confusion, or blurred vision. Fainting may occur. This condition is usually mild and may only last for a few minutes. Treatment is not required if this happens only occasionally. If the patient becomes unconscious for more than a few minutes, emergency medical treatment should be instituted. This may occur because of pregnancy, dehydration, heart issues, or diabetes. Pregnant women may experience a similar reaction when seated in the chair in a supine position because the uterus may be pressing on the abdominal veins. The woman should be positioned on her left side to allow improved blood flow.

**42. C:** Difficulty speaking, paralysis on one side of the body, sudden change in vision, or a sudden onset of a headache may be signs of a cerebrovascular accident or stroke. Other symptoms may include difficulty with walking, loss of coordination, or trouble finding words. Patients with a history of heart disease or uncontrolled hypertension are at risk. A simple test called FAST can be done to determine if this is a possibility. F is for face, A is for arms, S is for speech, and T is for time.

Ask the patient to smile (does one side of the face droop?), ask them to raise both arms over their head (does one arm slowly fall back down?), ask the patient to speak (is the speech slurred?), and call 911 immediately if any of these signs occur. Time is extremely important in stroke treatment. The best outcomes occur if treatment is given within the first 60 minutes of symptom occurrence.

**43. B:** Dry mouth, headache, and a fruity, acetone breath odor are all signs of hyperglycemia or elevated blood sugar. Other signs include excessive urination, blurred vision, rapid pulse, and decreased blood pressure. If untreated, it can lead to loss of consciousness. Type 1 diabetes is always treated with insulin. These patients are at risk for hyperglycemia as well as hypoglycemia. It is important to determine if the patient has eaten recently and if insulin was taken as ordered by his or her physician. In this case, the patient has not taken insulin and insulin administration is required immediately. If the patient has access to his or her insulin, assistance should be provided. Otherwise, alternative arrangements must be made to obtain insulin immediately, including calling the patient's emergency contact or 911 if necessary. Untreated short-term hyperglycemia can lead to serious complications that may require hospitalization.

**44. D:** Oral candidiasis is an infection in the mouth caused by a yeast-like fungus named *Candida albicans*. It is also known as oral thrush. Symptoms include creamy white lesions that look like cottage cheese on the tongue or inner cheeks but may also appear on the gums, roof of the mouth, and tonsils. The lesions may bleed when scraped. If the lesions spread to the esophagus, difficulty swallowing may result. Patients who have a weakened immune system, have diabetes, or are receiving antibiotic therapy are at risk for developing this condition. Oral candidiasis is treated with a topical antifungal medication, such as nystatin, taken in the form of a lozenge or a liquid that is swished around in the mouth then spit out.

**45. B:** Hepatitis B virus (HBV) is the cause of 34% of all acute viral hepatitis illnesses. Some people can be exposed to HBV but do not become ill. They can be carriers of this disease and unknowingly pass it along to others. Transmission is through blood and other types of bodily fluids including saliva. The Occupational Safety and Health Administration (OSHA) mandates that any employee who is starting a job that increases the chances of occupational exposure to HBV be offered the HBV vaccination within 10 days. The employee does not have to take advantage of this vaccination but must sign a release stating the vaccination was offered and the risks are understood. Other types of hepatitis include hepatitis A virus (HAV), which can infect anyone. It is spread through the fecal-oral route. Good handwashing is essential to prevent transmission of HAV. Hepatitis C virus (HCV) is mainly transmitted through blood and is generally contracted through use of contaminated needles.

**46. A:** Automatic shipments are a way for dental supplies to be ordered in bulk at a discounted rate. Only a portion of the order is shipped at a time, eliminating the need to find storage for a large bulk order. Supplies arrive periodically. Billing is also spread out over time, such as quarterly or monthly. Quantity purchase rate is also purchasing in bulk; however, typically the entire order must be received at one time. Ample storage space must be available for this type of ordering. Reorder quantity is the maximum amount of product that can be ordered at any one time and reflects frequency of use, shelf life, type of storage required, and availability of storage. Reorder point is the minimum quantity of a certain product that should be on hand at any one time. If the inventory goes below this number, the stock must be replenished.

**47. B:** Equipment records are important for keeping track of the model, serial number, date of purchase, and any servicing the equipment received. A service contract is critical to the smooth functioning of the dental office. If any of the key pieces of equipment break down, a service contract would help to ensure a quick response for emergency repair needs. Some service contracts will also include preventive routine maintenance. Manufacturer warranties are also important and typically cover repair or replacement for a certain length of time. Warranty information should be included as part of the equipment records. Another way to repair equipment is a service call. These tend to be expensive because the fee is based on mileage, amount of time required to repair, and the expertise of the technician. Service calls are typically used as a last resort. The cause of the issue should be explored thoroughly before making a service call, such as checking to make sure power is intact, check the reset button, or check the fuse box.

**48. A:** There are many different types of dental insurance. Each type may use a different method for calculating fees for service benefits, including fixed fee schedule, schedule of benefits, and UCR (usual, customary, and reasonable) fees. A deductible is the amount of money that must be paid towards the insurer's dental treatment before the insurance benefits will be activated. A copayment is the way dental treatment fees are split between the insurance carrier and the insured. Many carriers will split 80/20, where the insurance covers 80% and the insured must pay 20% of the total fee. Benefit eligibility is the term used to determine if the insured is able to start receiving benefits. New employees typically have to wait 30 to 60 days before benefits are activated. Many insurance carriers will require a pretreatment estimate or predetermination of benefits before any substantial dental work is initiated to make sure the patient and dentist are aware of the coverage that is available.

**49. D:** The state Dental Practice Act is a set of laws enacted by individual states to protect the public from dental providers who may not be fully qualified to practice. The legal requirements vary between each state but typically cover many of the same issues. It is important for dental assistants to be very familiar with the law in the state where they are practicing. Most of the state's Dental Practice Act is available for review on the internet. The Dental Practice Act typically includes requirements surrounding licensure and renewal of licenses. It sets the guidelines for appropriate level of continuing education that must be done over a specified time. It will specify the specific responsibilities that can be covered by dental assistants and dental hygienists. It will include rules and regulations surrounding the use of radiation and infection control.

**50. C:** The Health Insurance Portability and Accountability Act of 1996 (HIPAA) was enacted to help set national standards for the protection of health information. A dental office that transmits any health-related information electronically is required to comply with this law. This law also requires the development of a privacy policy for patients that must be reviewed with the patient and kept on file to acknowledge that the patient received and accepted the policy. Training for all personnel in the office is also required for safekeeping of patients' medical information. A policy regarding discipline of employees who breach patient privacy information is also required.

# How to Overcome Test Anxiety

Just the thought of taking a test is enough to make most people a little nervous. A test is an important event that can have a long-term impact on your future, so it's important to take it seriously and it's natural to feel anxious about performing well. But just because anxiety is normal, that doesn't mean that it's helpful in test taking, or that you should simply accept it as part of your life. Anxiety can have a variety of effects. These effects can be mild, like making you feel slightly nervous, or severe, like blocking your ability to focus or remember even a simple detail.

If you experience test anxiety—whether severe or mild—it's important to know how to beat it. To discover this, first you need to understand what causes test anxiety.

## Causes of Test Anxiety

While we often think of anxiety as an uncontrollable emotional state, it can actually be caused by simple, practical things. One of the most common causes of test anxiety is that a person does not feel adequately prepared for their test. This feeling can be the result of many different issues such as poor study habits or lack of organization, but the most common culprit is time management. Starting to study too late, failing to organize your study time to cover all of the material, or being distracted while you study will mean that you're not well prepared for the test. This may lead to cramming the night before, which will cause you to be physically and mentally exhausted for the test. Poor time management also contributes to feelings of stress, fear, and hopelessness as you realize you are not well prepared but don't know what to do about it.

Other times, test anxiety is not related to your preparation for the test but comes from unresolved fear. This may be a past failure on a test, or poor performance on tests in general. It may come from comparing yourself to others who seem to be performing better or from the stress of living up to expectations. Anxiety may be driven by fears of the future—how failure on this test would affect your educational and career goals. These fears are often completely irrational, but they can still negatively impact your test performance.

> **Review Video: 3 Reasons You Have Test Anxiety**
> Visit mometrix.com/academy and enter code: 428468

# Elements of Test Anxiety

As mentioned earlier, test anxiety is considered to be an emotional state, but it has physical and mental components as well. Sometimes you may not even realize that you are suffering from test anxiety until you notice the physical symptoms. These can include trembling hands, rapid heartbeat, sweating, nausea, and tense muscles. Extreme anxiety may lead to fainting or vomiting. Obviously, any of these symptoms can have a negative impact on testing. It is important to recognize them as soon as they begin to occur so that you can address the problem before it damages your performance.

> **Review Video: 3 Ways to Tell You Have Test Anxiety**
> Visit mometrix.com/academy and enter code: 927847

The mental components of test anxiety include trouble focusing and inability to remember learned information. During a test, your mind is on high alert, which can help you recall information and stay focused for an extended period of time. However, anxiety interferes with your mind's natural processes, causing you to blank out, even on the questions you know well. The strain of testing during anxiety makes it difficult to stay focused, especially on a test that may take several hours. Extreme anxiety can take a huge mental toll, making it difficult not only to recall test information but even to understand the test questions or pull your thoughts together.

> **Review Video: How Test Anxiety Affects Memory**
> Visit mometrix.com/academy and enter code: 609003

# Effects of Test Anxiety

Test anxiety is like a disease—if left untreated, it will get progressively worse. Anxiety leads to poor performance, and this reinforces the feelings of fear and failure, which in turn lead to poor performances on subsequent tests. It can grow from a mild nervousness to a crippling condition. If allowed to progress, test anxiety can have a big impact on your schooling, and consequently on your future.

Test anxiety can spread to other parts of your life. Anxiety on tests can become anxiety in any stressful situation, and blanking on a test can turn into panicking in a job situation. But fortunately, you don't have to let anxiety rule your testing and determine your grades. There are a number of relatively simple steps you can take to move past anxiety and function normally on a test and in the rest of life.

> **Review Video: How Test Anxiety Impacts Your Grades**
> Visit mometrix.com/academy and enter code: 939819

# Physical Steps for Beating Test Anxiety

While test anxiety is a serious problem, the good news is that it can be overcome. It doesn't have to control your ability to think and remember information. While it may take time, you can begin taking steps today to beat anxiety.

Just as your first hint that you may be struggling with anxiety comes from the physical symptoms, the first step to treating it is also physical. Rest is crucial for having a clear, strong mind. If you are tired, it is much easier to give in to anxiety. But if you establish good sleep habits, your body and mind will be ready to perform optimally, without the strain of exhaustion. Additionally, sleeping well helps you to retain information better, so you're more likely to recall the answers when you see the test questions.

Getting good sleep means more than going to bed on time. It's important to allow your brain time to relax. Take study breaks from time to time so it doesn't get overworked, and don't study right before bed. Take time to rest your mind before trying to rest your body, or you may find it difficult to fall asleep.

> **Review Video: The Importance of Sleep for Your Brain**
> Visit mometrix.com/academy and enter code: 319338

Along with sleep, other aspects of physical health are important in preparing for a test. Good nutrition is vital for good brain function. Sugary foods and drinks may give a burst of energy but this burst is followed by a crash, both physically and emotionally. Instead, fuel your body with protein and vitamin-rich foods.

Also, drink plenty of water. Dehydration can lead to headaches and exhaustion, especially if your brain is already under stress from the rigors of the test. Particularly if your test is a long one, drink water during the breaks. And if possible, take an energy-boosting snack to eat between sections.

> **Review Video: How Diet Can Affect your Mood**
> Visit mometrix.com/academy and enter code: 624317

Along with sleep and diet, a third important part of physical health is exercise. Maintaining a steady workout schedule is helpful, but even taking 5-minute study breaks to walk can help get your blood pumping faster and clear your head. Exercise also releases endorphins, which contribute to a positive feeling and can help combat test anxiety.

When you nurture your physical health, you are also contributing to your mental health. If your body is healthy, your mind is much more likely to be healthy as well. So take time to rest, nourish your body with healthy food and water, and get moving as much as possible. Taking these physical steps will make you stronger and more able to take the mental steps necessary to overcome test anxiety.

# Mental Steps for Beating Test Anxiety

Working on the mental side of test anxiety can be more challenging, but as with the physical side, there are clear steps you can take to overcome it. As mentioned earlier, test anxiety often stems from lack of preparation, so the obvious solution is to prepare for the test. Effective studying may be the most important weapon you have for beating test anxiety, but you can and should employ several other mental tools to combat fear.

First, boost your confidence by reminding yourself of past success—tests or projects that you aced. If you're putting as much effort into preparing for this test as you did for those, there's no reason you should expect to fail here. Work hard to prepare; then trust your preparation.

Second, surround yourself with encouraging people. It can be helpful to find a study group, but be sure that the people you're around will encourage a positive attitude. If you spend time with others who are anxious or cynical, this will only contribute to your own anxiety. Look for others who are motivated to study hard from a desire to succeed, not from a fear of failure.

Third, reward yourself. A test is physically and mentally tiring, even without anxiety, and it can be helpful to have something to look forward to. Plan an activity following the test, regardless of the outcome, such as going to a movie or getting ice cream.

When you are taking the test, if you find yourself beginning to feel anxious, remind yourself that you know the material. Visualize successfully completing the test. Then take a few deep, relaxing breaths and return to it. Work through the questions carefully but with confidence, knowing that you are capable of succeeding.

Developing a healthy mental approach to test taking will also aid in other areas of life. Test anxiety affects more than just the actual test—it can be damaging to your mental health and even contribute to depression. It's important to beat test anxiety before it becomes a problem for more than testing.

> **Review Video: Test Anxiety and Depression**
> Visit mometrix.com/academy and enter code: 904704

# Study Strategy

Being prepared for the test is necessary to combat anxiety, but what does being prepared look like? You may study for hours on end and still not feel prepared. What you need is a strategy for test prep. The next few pages outline our recommended steps to help you plan out and conquer the challenge of preparation.

## STEP 1: SCOPE OUT THE TEST

Learn everything you can about the format (multiple choice, essay, etc.) and what will be on the test. Gather any study materials, course outlines, or sample exams that may be available. Not only will this help you to prepare, but knowing what to expect can help to alleviate test anxiety.

## STEP 2: MAP OUT THE MATERIAL

Look through the textbook or study guide and make note of how many chapters or sections it has. Then divide these over the time you have. For example, if a book has 15 chapters and you have five days to study, you need to cover three chapters each day. Even better, if you have the time, leave an extra day at the end for overall review after you have gone through the material in depth.

If time is limited, you may need to prioritize the material. Look through it and make note of which sections you think you already have a good grasp on, and which need review. While you are studying, skim quickly through the familiar sections and take more time on the challenging parts. Write out your plan so you don't get lost as you go. Having a written plan also helps you feel more in control of the study, so anxiety is less likely to arise from feeling overwhelmed at the amount to cover.

## STEP 3: GATHER YOUR TOOLS

Decide what study method works best for you. Do you prefer to highlight in the book as you study and then go back over the highlighted portions? Or do you type out notes of the important information? Or is it helpful to make flashcards that you can carry with you? Assemble the pens, index cards, highlighters, post-it notes, and any other materials you may need so you won't be distracted by getting up to find things while you study.

If you're having a hard time retaining the information or organizing your notes, experiment with different methods. For example, try color-coding by subject with colored pens, highlighters, or post-it notes. If you learn better by hearing, try recording yourself reading your notes so you can listen while in the car, working out, or simply sitting at your desk. Ask a friend to quiz you from your flashcards, or try teaching someone the material to solidify it in your mind.

## STEP 4: CREATE YOUR ENVIRONMENT

It's important to avoid distractions while you study. This includes both the obvious distractions like visitors and the subtle distractions like an uncomfortable chair (or a too-comfortable couch that makes you want to fall asleep). Set up the best study environment possible: good lighting and a comfortable work area. If background music helps you focus, you may want to turn it on, but otherwise keep the room quiet. If you are using a computer to take notes, be sure you don't have any other windows open, especially applications like social media, games, or anything else that could distract you. Silence your phone and turn off notifications. Be sure to keep water close by so you stay hydrated while you study (but avoid unhealthy drinks and snacks).

Also, take into account the best time of day to study. Are you freshest first thing in the morning? Try to set aside some time then to work through the material. Is your mind clearer in the afternoon or evening? Schedule your study session then. Another method is to study at the same time of day that you will take the test, so that your brain gets used to working on the material at that time and will be ready to focus at test time.

## STEP 5: STUDY!

Once you have done all the study preparation, it's time to settle into the actual studying. Sit down, take a few moments to settle your mind so you can focus, and begin to follow your study plan. Don't give in to distractions or let yourself procrastinate. This is your time to prepare so you'll be ready to fearlessly approach the test. Make the most of the time and stay focused.

Of course, you don't want to burn out. If you study too long you may find that you're not retaining the information very well. Take regular study breaks. For example, taking five minutes out of every hour to walk briskly, breathing deeply and swinging your arms, can help your mind stay fresh.

As you get to the end of each chapter or section, it's a good idea to do a quick review. Remind yourself of what you learned and work on any difficult parts. When you feel that you've mastered the material, move on to the next part. At the end of your study session, briefly skim through your notes again.

But while review is helpful, cramming last minute is NOT. If at all possible, work ahead so that you won't need to fit all your study into the last day. Cramming overloads your brain with more information than it can process and retain, and your tired mind may struggle to recall even previously learned information when it is overwhelmed with last-minute study. Also, the urgent nature of cramming and the stress placed on your brain contribute to anxiety. You'll be more likely to go to the test feeling unprepared and having trouble thinking clearly.

So don't cram, and don't stay up late before the test, even just to review your notes at a leisurely pace. Your brain needs rest more than it needs to go over the information again. In fact, plan to finish your studies by noon or early afternoon the day before the test. Give your brain the rest of the day to relax or focus on other things, and get a good night's sleep. Then you will be fresh for the test and better able to recall what you've studied.

## STEP 6: TAKE A PRACTICE TEST

Many courses offer sample tests, either online or in the study materials. This is an excellent resource to check whether you have mastered the material, as well as to prepare for the test format and environment.

Check the test format ahead of time: the number of questions, the type (multiple choice, free response, etc.), and the time limit. Then create a plan for working through them. For example, if you have 30 minutes to take a 60-question test, your limit is 30 seconds per question. Spend less time on the questions you know well so that you can take more time on the difficult ones.

If you have time to take several practice tests, take the first one open book, with no time limit. Work through the questions at your own pace and make sure you fully understand them. Gradually work up to taking a test under test conditions: sit at a desk with all study materials put away and set a timer. Pace yourself to make sure you finish the test with time to spare and go back to check your answers if you have time.

After each test, check your answers. On the questions you missed, be sure you understand why you missed them. Did you misread the question (tests can use tricky wording)? Did you forget the information? Or was it something you hadn't learned? Go back and study any shaky areas that the practice tests reveal.

Taking these tests not only helps with your grade, but also aids in combating test anxiety. If you're already used to the test conditions, you're less likely to worry about it, and working through tests until you're scoring well gives you a confidence boost. Go through the practice tests until you feel comfortable, and then you can go into the test knowing that you're ready for it.

## Test Tips

On test day, you should be confident, knowing that you've prepared well and are ready to answer the questions. But aside from preparation, there are several test day strategies you can employ to maximize your performance.

First, as stated before, get a good night's sleep the night before the test (and for several nights before that, if possible). Go into the test with a fresh, alert mind rather than staying up late to study.

Try not to change too much about your normal routine on the day of the test. It's important to eat a nutritious breakfast, but if you normally don't eat breakfast at all, consider eating just a protein bar. If you're a coffee drinker, go ahead and have your normal coffee. Just make sure you time it so that the caffeine doesn't wear off right in the middle of your test. Avoid sugary beverages, and drink enough water to stay hydrated but not so much that you need a restroom break 10 minutes into the test. If your test isn't first thing in the morning, consider going for a walk or doing a light workout before the test to get your blood flowing.

Allow yourself enough time to get ready, and leave for the test with plenty of time to spare so you won't have the anxiety of scrambling to arrive in time. Another reason to be early is to select a good seat. It's helpful to sit away from doors and windows, which can be distracting. Find a good seat, get out your supplies, and settle your mind before the test begins.

When the test begins, start by going over the instructions carefully, even if you already know what to expect. Make sure you avoid any careless mistakes by following the directions.

Then begin working through the questions, pacing yourself as you've practiced. If you're not sure on an answer, don't spend too much time on it, and don't let it shake your confidence. Either skip it and come back later, or eliminate as many wrong answers as possible and guess among the remaining ones. Don't dwell on these questions as you continue—put them out of your mind and focus on what lies ahead.

Be sure to read all of the answer choices, even if you're sure the first one is the right answer. Sometimes you'll find a better one if you keep reading. But don't second-guess yourself if you do immediately know the answer. Your gut instinct is usually right. Don't let test anxiety rob you of the information you know.

If you have time at the end of the test (and if the test format allows), go back and review your answers. Be cautious about changing any, since your first instinct tends to be correct, but make sure you didn't misread any of the questions or accidentally mark the wrong answer choice. Look over any you skipped and make an educated guess.

At the end, leave the test feeling confident. You've done your best, so don't waste time worrying about your performance or wishing you could change anything. Instead, celebrate the successful completion of this test. And finally, use this test to learn how to deal with anxiety even better next time.

## Important Qualification

Not all anxiety is created equal. If your test anxiety is causing major issues in your life beyond the classroom or testing center, or if you are experiencing troubling physical symptoms related to your anxiety, it may be a sign of a serious physiological or psychological condition. If this sounds like your situation, we strongly encourage you to seek professional help.

# Thank You

We at Mometrix would like to extend our heartfelt thanks to you, our friend and patron, for allowing us to play a part in your journey. It is a privilege to serve people from all walks of life who are unified in their commitment to building the best future they can for themselves.

The preparation you devote to these important testing milestones may be the most valuable educational opportunity you have for making a real difference in your life. We encourage you to put your heart into it—that feeling of succeeding, overcoming, and yes, conquering will be well worth the hours you've invested.

We want to hear your story, your struggles and your successes, and if you see any opportunities for us to improve our materials so we can help others even more effectively in the future, please share that with us as well. **The team at Mometrix would be absolutely thrilled to hear from you!** So please, send us an email (support@mometrix.com) and let's stay in touch.

> **If you'd like some additional help, check out these other resources we offer for your exam:**
> http://mometrixflashcards.com/DANB

# Additional Bonus Material

Due to our efforts to try to keep this book to a manageable length, we've created a link that will give you access to all of your additional bonus material:

**mometrix.com/bonus948/danbgc**